the Marie Antoinette diet

EAT CAKE
AND STILL
LOSE WEIGHT

KAREN WHEELER

Consultant Dietician: Dr Mabel Blades

SP

Sweet Pea Publishing

First published as an Ebook by Sweet Pea Publishing in 2013

Cover photograph © Klenova | Dreamstime.com

A catalogue record for this book is available from the British library.

ISBN: 978-0-9571066-5-9

Sweet Pea Publishing
PO Box 67770,
London, W14 4EF

www.sweetpeapublishing.com

Typeset by Bookcraft Ltd, Stroud, Gloucestershire
Printed in Great Britain by CPI Group Ltd, Croydon CR0 4YY

For my grandparents, Mary and Harry Wheeler

(and cake lovers everywhere)

CONTENTS

IMPORTANT NOTE

The author is not a medical or scientific expert and does not claim to be. The information contained in this book is intended for general purposes only and should not be relied upon as a substitute for medical advice, diagnosis or treatment.

As with any diet, be sure to consult your doctor before adopting this eating plan or acting on any of the information in this book. This is especially important if you are pregnant, diabetic, have existing heart, cardiovascular or other health problems or are taking any kind of medication.

Vegetarians should also note that although the Marie Antoinette Diet can easily be adapted, it is not particularly vegetarian-friendly, although many of the recipes are delicious and contain no meat. Those on the intermittent fasting diet may also find the advice in the book useful, and the soup recipes ideal for fasting days.

This is not a fad diet but rather a healthy way of eating, designed for sustainable weight loss. Although it is possible to lose over a kilo or several pounds in a week, without excluding any food groups and eating normally most of the day, it does assume a degree of moderation. If you are regularly ploughing through a big helping of Black Forest gateau, or even several portions of the cakes featured within these pages, the diet will not result in magical weight loss.

Finally, the author has made every effort to check available facts and the most up-to-date research, but neither she nor the publisher or anyone involved in the book's production, will be liable for any injury, harm or other consequences or claims resulting from the use or misuse of information, suggestions or scientific research quoted within these pages, or any errors, omissions or misinformation, including that which might come to light as a result of subsequent research.

The author and publisher will however, share the delight of readers who lose weight and improve their health as a result of the Marie Antoinette Diet.

ABOUT ME

In my former life, I was the fashion editor of *The Mail on Sunday* newspaper in the UK, and subsequently, the beauty and lifestyle editor of a health and beauty magazine. As a freelance, I edited the health and well-being section of *The London Magazine* for five years, where I worked with many alternative therapists and learned a lot about nutrition and the use of food as medicine.

I also wrote on beauty and anti-aging, among other subjects, for *The Financial Times How To Spend It* magazine for over a decade. And prior to all of this, I studied modern history at King's College, London University, where I acquired an enduring interest in 18th-century France and Marie Antoinette.

In my late thirties, I moved to France myself, wrote three travel memoirs and gained over 10 kilos (1st 8lb) in three years. Of the many diets I'd encountered during my career, none seemed remotely appealing or doable when I needed to lose weight myself. But if I wasn't to spend the rest of my life in smock tops and large prints, I had to find a way of losing the surplus poundage as painlessly as possible. It would, I realized, have to be a diet that didn't involve counting calories, deprivation, or eating cocktail sausages for breakfast, as friends on high-protein diets have done. Almost by chance, I created a diet that worked for me, resulting in fairly effortless weight loss while eating normally most of the time. I hope that others with a weakness for cake will find it useful too. Finally, as already stated, I'm not a dietician but because I wanted the Marie Antoinette Diet to be as safe and effective as possible, I consulted someone who is:

Dr MABEL BLADES

Dr Mabel Blades BSC RD is a registered dietician and nutritionist and an expert in the treatment of disorders by diet. A member of the British Dietetic Association, her work includes food consultancy, recipe development and teaching, as well as research and lecturing. She is the former editor of *Nutrition and Food Science* and has written numerous papers and articles as well as a book on nutrition and health. Dr Blades, whose PhD focused on diabetes, has checked the nutritional advice in this book, to ensure that the diet is safe to follow.

ABOUT THE SCIENCE

We are bombarded with so much contradictory information regarding food, diet and health that it is difficult to know what to believe. When I started researching this book, I quickly realized that for every study saying one thing, there is another saying the exact opposite. It is very easy to support a theory by cherry-picking the relevant piece of science. For this reason, I've tried to flag up where the research I've cited is flawed in any way, or contradicted by other studies. That way, readers get the wider picture and can ultimately decide for themselves. Also, whenever a piece of scientific research is quoted, this means that I have actually read it – or at least, in a few cases, an abstract from it – rather than just rehashing it from the Internet. For as I also discovered, quite a lot of the information that is out there, including the nutritional claims made for various foods, is erroneous.

PART ONE

INTRODUCTION

The wake-up call

For most of my adult life I have worked in fashion, and for all of my adult life, I have loved cake. Yet reconciling my passion for cream-filled éclairs, macaroons and chocolate cake with a career where skinny hips are mandatory, proved surprisingly easy. Somehow, the calories were burned off as nervous energy as I ran around Paris, Milan and New York to meetings in my high-rise heels and (UK) size 10 skirts.

Then I gave up my city life and moved to France to become a full-time writer. I loved my new lifestyle. But as the stress melted away, so the weight started to creep up. A combination of hitting my forties, constant access to the fridge and the fact that I was no longer running around to meetings – or even walking to the office water cooler – meant that the pounds piled on.

I like food, I never say 'no' to dessert and I'm fond of a glass of wine with dinner. Since moving to the land of the long lunch, I had indulged freely in all the croissants, patisserie and fine red wines that France had to offer. Much of the social life in France revolves around eating enormous meals in other peoples' houses, while in the winter months it is easy to fall into the trap of closing the shutters, lighting the fire and cooking a calorie-laden dinner, before collapsing on the sofa with a glass of wine for the rest of the evening.

The wake-up call came, as it does for many people, in the form of a photograph. In the Dordogne for a book signing last summer, my niece took a photo of me looking out of a window with my little dog Biff standing on his hind legs beside me. It was a really sweet picture. Just one problem: the rear view couldn't possibly be mine. It didn't chime with my perception of myself as a fairly svelte (UK) size 10–12.

I even began to wonder if I was suffering from the opposite of body dysmorphic disorder, the condition in which sufferers imagine themselves to be overweight when they are not, or so-called 'fat blindness', the recently coined phrase for people who ignore weight gain. Either way, here was the visible proof that I was no longer the reasonably slim person that I had always been.

I weighed 62kg (9st 10.7lb) when I left London; in France, the scales at one point tipped a sobering 75kg (11st 11lb). The ideal weight for someone of my height of 5'6", is

53 to 70kg (8st 5lb to 11st 1lb). And so it became my mission to drop at least 10kg (1st 8lb) to return to something like my former weight.

The problem was not immediately apparent because, in my previous life as a fashion editor, I'd learned a few tricks to disguise surplus poundage. Most of the excess had piled on around my middle – the most dangerous place since fat there is visceral or unseen fat, wrapped around your internal organs, and it is linked with diabetes, cardiovascular disease and (oh triple woe!) dementia.[1] But as I had discovered, a smock top or a big cardigan over skinny jeans could disguise at least five of those extra ten kilos.

Expert as I was at hiding the evidence, I didn't like how I felt – sluggish and lacking in energy, especially in the mornings. With hindsight, it is perhaps understandable if your body doesn't want to get out of bed first thing when it knows that it will be lugging the equivalent of an extra ten bags of sugar around all day. I also noticed that my energy slumped dramatically in the mid-afternoon.

The second wake-up call came when I went for a medical check up and my doctor expressed concern about my waist size, which had increased to an alarming 89cm (35 inches). Traditionally, diabetes experts have used the BMI or body mass index calculation, of weight related to height, to assess risk of diabetes but as my doctor pointed out, there is also a strong link between waist size and the likelihood of contracting diabetes.

A study that evaluated data on more than 28,500 people in eight European countries found that women whose waists measure 89cm (35 inches) or more, and men with a waist measurement over 101cm (40 inches), have a risk of diabetes equal to that of obese people.[2] High waist size was a stronger risk factor for women than for men. Obese women with a waist over 89cm (35 inches) meanwhile, were nearly 32 times more likely to get diabetes than women in the low to normal weight range, with a waist of less than 79cm (31 inches). I listened as my doctor gave me these sobering statistics, and left the surgery determined that something had to be done. But what?

Diets are a drag (and some are dangerous)

Diet books are a drag. They tell you to eat carrot batons and cucumber sticks instead of chocolate when that mid-afternoon sugar craving hits. Like that's going to work. As for extreme slimming regimes, the faster you lose weight, the more quickly you seem to put it back on again; while the continual sense of denial makes it almost inevitable that you will eventually succumb to a bout of binge eating.

During my career as a fashion journalist, I saw many fad diets come and go. On my bookshelves is a beauty bible from the 1970s, produced by a well-known magazine, which I consult whenever I want to be reminded of the folly of crash diets. It proposes in all seriousness, the 'Drinker's Diet' (a seven day plan that allows you two drinks of whisky, gin or vodka with lunch and dinner) and the 'Wine and Eggs Diet' (three days of either cheese or three hard boiled eggs, washed down by a bottle of white wine a day – 'dry, preferably Chablis'!) Presumably you are so nauseated by the idea of yet another boiled egg, or so sozzled by the alcohol, that you can't face the thought of eating anything. Still, they all sound marginally less loony than the 'HCG Diet Plan' outlined in the same book and based on daily injections of human chorionic gonadotropin (HCG), a hormone obtained from the urine of pregnant women.

With the benefit of three decades of hindsight, these diets seem horrifying and hilarious in equal measure. I'm convinced that some years from now, we'll view many of today's fashionable diets with equal scepticism. That's not to say that I didn't consider them. Many people, I know, have lost weight through high-protein, no-carb diets, but along with many medical experts, I cannot believe that such regimes are good for the body. Too much protein puts the liver and kidneys under strain, as they struggle to process the by-products of protein metabolism. Other side effects are said to include constipation, low blood pressure and a general feeling of malaise – not exactly a dream ticket to weight loss.

I was also attracted by the concept of intermittent fasting – a diet that is currently hugely popular in the UK, and through which many people have lost weight. The idea that you can eat anything you want for five days of the week, so long as you limit calorie intake for the other two, seemed very attractive. I liked the fact that fasting gets the thumbs up from members of the medical profession, that it has been practiced by many cultures for centuries, and that research has shown it to reduce the risk of diabetes and cardiovascular disease[3] and boost longevity. It sounded like an all-round winner – until I tried it.

On the fasting day, when calorie intake is restricted to 500 for women, 600 for men, not only did I feel 'hangry' (a combination of 'hungry' and 'angry' caused by low blood sugar) but also light-headed and unable to focus. After blowing a large chunk of my calorie allowance on a morning bowl of porridge with a dash of maple syrup, the hunger gnawed away until no longer possible to ignore, culminating in a hastily fried egg and chips at midnight.

The conclusion: it might work for many other people – and I'm not knocking it, as I can also see the health benefits of giving the digestive system a rest – but for me to adhere to this diet, I would need to be anaesthetized for the fasting day.

However, I liked the simplicity of intermittent fasting and the fact that it didn't involve counting calories or following complicated meal plans. In order to lose my ten kilos, I needed to find an equally simple regime – one that did not ban any food groups, since nothing is guaranteed to make me want something more than knowing that I can't have it. In order for me to stick with it, the ideal weight loss plan would have to be healthy and include some fruit and lots of vegetables, but it would also have to leave scope for a little naughtiness.

French women eat cake

How French women stay slim, while routinely navigating three or four richly calorific courses at mealtimes, has long been a subject of debate. Many theories have been put forward, from plain old portion control to excessive intake of nicotine. Having lived in France for seven years, I was well placed to observe at close quarters the cunning ways in which French women stay thin. Unfortunately, with the exception of a few acquaintances who appeared to survive on a diet of caffeine, green salad and nicotine, there had been no blinding revelation, no single magic trick that I had observed that would allow me to indulge freely in all the delights that France had to offer, and still fit my clothes.

But I had noticed one thing: French women do eat cake. And bread. And butter. And fat-filled pâtés. It is true that French women do not, in general, drink much alcohol, which would account for some calorie saving. So too, would portion control – the French eat rich, fatty and highly-flavoured food, but they do so in small amounts – and the fact that snacks between meals are regarded (*quelle horreur!*), as a kind of uncouth gluttony. But there had to be another secret strategy, an unspoken 'French Women Don't Get Fat Plan' that the sisterhood *française* did not want to share with the rest of the world. French women, I've noticed, never talk about dieting or the need to lose weight. When I asked around among slim French friends, I was given the usual Gallic shrug and told that the secret was to 'eat less' or that 'the best way to lose weight is to have problems in love'. (Interestingly, a recent survey suggests that having an affair can also lead to weight loss.[4])

It was while reading a biography of Marie Antoinette that the light bulb moment occurred (and before you ask, the solution to weight gain does not lie in having your head chopped off). In *Marie Antoinette*, the movie, director Sofia Coppola depicted the French Queen's life as one long cake-fest, gorging on macaroons and fondant-filled pastries, washed down with a river of champagne. It is true that Marie Antoinette had a sweet tooth. It is also true that she was no saint. She had coffee or hot chocolate for breakfast, accompanied by a pastry, which was, in all likelihood, an early version of the croissant. This was not the only temptation put in her way. The court of Versailles, in the years running up to the Revolution, was renowned for its extravagance and lavish cuisine. During Louis XIV's reign, a formal meal would be divided into a number of 'services' including hors d'oeuvres, soups, and main courses. Within each service there would be between two and eight dishes, which for an official dinner, could amount to up to thirty dishes in a sitting.

These formal dinners had become more restrained by the time Marie Antoinette and her husband, Louis XVI, ascended the throne, with rich, heavily-spiced dishes giving way to simpler fare or *le goût naturel*.[5] But the court cuisine continued to be calorific and abundant: typically, pâté in pastry, oysters, lobster, langoustines or other crustacea for hors d'oeuvres, followed by opulent main courses such as hare stew, roast beef, scallops, duck, salmon, fish in buttery sauces or breaded foie gras with rice, and then a selection of lighter entremets or 'between courses' that were thought to soothe the stomach. According to Susan Pinkard, author of *A Revolution In Taste: the Rise of French Cuisine, 1650–1800*, examples of these 'lighter' dishes included cheese and cooked egg recipes, foods in aspic, fritters and pastries, macaroni, and vegetables fricasseed in cream. *Not exactly crudités and salad, then.* Next came the desserts: milk or cream-based dishes such as custards, rice pudding and blancmange were popular at the time, as were fresh cream cheeses served with sugar. And in a final flurry of calories, the dessert course would often be accompanied by a selection of biscuits, wafers, delicate pastries, fruits (both crystallized and fresh), and petits fours.

Faced with such an onslaught of temptation and rich food, how did Marie Antoinette stay slim? At Versailles there would have been some powerful appetite suppressants working in her favour, including the smell of the palace. Versailles, at the time, lacked modern plumbing, and it was quite normal for people to squat down wherever and whenever the bodily urge took them. As Marie Antoinette's perfumer Jean-Louis Fargeon wrote of his first visit there, 'The park, the gardens, even the chateau, turn the stomach with their dreadful odours. The hallways, the courtyards, the buildings and corridors are filled with urine and faecal matter.'

Court customs would also have curbed the appetite. 'One of the customs most disagreeable to the Queen was that of dining every day in public,' wrote Madame Campan, Marie Antoinette's confidante and first-lady-in-waiting, in her memoirs.[6] The Queen is said to have eaten nothing at these public meals, preferring to have lunch in private. Dressing and undressing in front of an audience, as Marie Antoinette was required to do daily before her noble-women, would also have provided motivation to keep her waist a trim 58cm (23 inches), the measurement recorded by her seamstress, Madame Éloffe.

Portraits of Marie Antoinette invariably depicted her with a tiny waist – and according to Caroline Weber, author of *Queen of Fashion: What Marie Antoinette Wore to the Revolution*, the Queen was slim enough to wear her formal gowns without the stiff whalebone corsets that were compulsory at the French court. Although Marie Antoinette did grow stouter after the birth of her children, forcing her to return to the stiff whalebone stays later in life, her waist was still small by today's standards. It was certainly below the 89cm (35 inches) that delineates the diabetes danger zone.

As was the custom of the 18th-century French court, the Queen would have eaten her main meal at lunchtime, usually served between noon and 3.00 pm. In the evening, she was noted to be very abstemious. Dinner, according to Madame Campan, would consist of a light broth and white meat – either a piece of chicken or guinea fowl – accompanied by vegetables from the well-stocked royal garden at Versailles. 'In the evening they always brought the Queen a large bowl of broth, a cold roast fowl, one bottle of wine, one of orgeat (a sweet syrup made from almonds, sugar and rose or orange flower water), one of lemonade, and some other articles, which were called the *en-cas*, or 'in case', for the night,' wrote Madame Campan.

It's possible that Marie Antoinette was herself following a diet of sorts. In the 18th century, food and medicine were closely linked. Among the genteel classes in England during the 1730s and 1740s, it was fashionable to follow a regime created by a Scottish-born physician, George Cheyne. To improve the health and remedy various ailments, Cheyne preached abstinence and devised a series of 'lowering' diets, gradually eliminating meats and fish. In *An Essay of Health and Long Life*, he argued that white and pale-coloured meats were healthier and 'lighter to digest, than those whose substance is redder, browner, or inclining towards the more flaming colours.' According to his theory, chicken, turkey, veal and rabbit were healthier than deep-red meats such as duck, woodcock, lamb and beef.

A version of Cheyne's diet eventually caught on in France – the philosopher Jean-Jacques Rousseau advocated a similar regime of simple flavours and frugal eating – and Marie Antoinette's focus on white meat suggests that she may have been influenced by it. Either way, contrary to the over-the-top indulgence portrayed in the Coppola movie, Marie Antoinette was teetotal and, sugar-rush breakfast aside, actually very restrained as far as food was concerned.

But restraint is not the whole story. The Queen liked sweet things, especially chocolate, pastry and water flavoured with sugary syrups, but Madame Campan's memoirs suggest that Marie Antoinette instinctively knew what 21st-century science has shown – namely, that it is not what you eat, but when you eat it. And the more I looked into the Queen's diet, the more I became convinced that it held the key to the so-called 'French paradox' – the question of how the French eat rich, fatty food yet still manage to stay slim and avoid coronary heart disease.

PART TWO

THE THEORY

1. Timing counts (and if you're going to eat cake, it's best to do so early in the day)

'Eat breakfast like a queen, lunch like a princess, and dinner like a pauperess,' so the saying (roughly) goes. Marie Antoinette's breakfast would be frowned upon by modern-day nutritionists, consisting as it did of carbs and caffeine (a croissant-like cake and either coffee or thick, gloopy hot chocolate, infused with her favourite orange blossom). There is a stack of research cataloguing the negative effects of sugar, and I won't go into it here, but recent studies suggest that if you are going to succumb to the sweet stuff, it may be better to do so early in the day.

Researchers at Vanderbilt University in Nashville recently established that insulin action in mice follows a 24-hour cycle and that the metabolism of fat and carbohydrate fluctuates throughout that period.[7] The study found that if mice ate food at a time when they would normally be inactive (that means during the day, since mice are nocturnal), the glucose was more likely to be stored as fat. Calories consumed during the time when mice are normally active, on the other hand, were more likely to be burned as energy or used for tissue building.

Although mice are nocturnal, on a molecular level their internal body clock is very similar to that of humans. As a result, the Vanderbilt scientists believe that humans would also benefit from timing their meals according to peaks in insulin efficiency. This would mean eating their main meal at lunchtime and a lighter meal in the evening – just as Marie Antoinette ate – while avoiding post-dinner snacks. 'Our study confirms that it is not only what you eat and how much you eat that is important for a healthy lifestyle, but when you eat is also very important,' said one of the researchers, Shu-qun Shi.

'The biological clock controls our metabolism, so the way in which we metabolize the same foods during the day and night is different,' explained Professor Carl Johnson, who led the study. 'If you metabolize food during the day, when you are active, you tend not to convert so much of that to fat. Whereas food eaten during the night or late evening is more likely to be converted into fat.' As a result of the findings, Professor Johnson declared that, 'Mediterranean diets, in which the main meal is eaten in the middle of the day are probably healthier.'

More research on humans is needed to prove the theory conclusively, but another study at Tel Aviv University also suggests that morning is the optimum time of day to eat cake.[8] The researchers split 193 clinically obese women into two groups. One group ate a low-carb diet with a 300-calorie breakfast, while the other enjoyed a balanced 600-calorie breakfast that included a chocolate cake for dessert. Those who ate the more calorific breakfast, featuring the chocolate cake, lost more weight on average than the participants who had a 300-calorie low-carb breakfast. Although both groups consumed the same daily amount of calories – the men 1600 calories per day and the women 1400 – at the end of the 32-week study, those who had consumed the 600-calorie, cake-inclusive breakfast had lost an average of 18kg (40lb) more per person than those in the other group. They also reported fewer cravings and were more successful at keeping the weight off.

The researchers concluded that eating a breakfast that includes cookies or chocolate, along with proteins and carbs, could help curb cravings for sweets later in the day. Professor Daniela Jakubowicz reported that, 'The participants in the low-carbohydrate diet group had less satisfaction and felt that they were not full.' As a result, their cravings for sugar and carbohydrate eventually led them to cheat on the diet plan. This suggests what many dieters already know: that restrictive diets that ban desserts and sweet treats are doomed to failure, because eventually you give in to cravings.

Eating a higher proportion of your daily calories at breakfast also makes sense because it kick-starts the metabolism and brain function. Professor Jakubowicz further pointed out that breakfast is the meal that most effectively suppresses ghrelin, the hormone that stimulates hunger, sending a signal to the brain that it is time to eat. This is important, as curbing cravings and the desire for food, is the key to successful slimming. (One of the reasons why high-protein diets lead to weight loss is that proteins induce a feeling of satiety or fullness.) The conclusion: early morning is the best time of day to eat cake. This is when the body's metabolism is most active, and as part of a balanced breakfast, it can actually encourage weight loss and maintenance, by keeping cravings in check. It helps too, that you then have the rest of the day to work off the calories.

2. A 12-hour nightly fast can help promote weight loss

The benefits of fasting and resting the digestive system have been recognized for centuries. In addition to weight loss, fasting has also been shown to reduce blood sugar and the risk of cancer. Recently, there has been much emphasis on the benefits of intermittent fasting, whereby you give up food or severely restrict calorie intake for a period of 24 hours, once or twice a week. But some experts believe that fasting overnight might have similar benefits.

As a result of the aforementioned study on mice at Vanderbilt University, Professor Johnson concluded that it might be a good idea 'to fast every day ... not eat anything between dinner and breakfast.' This echoes the findings of other research. In a study carried out at the Salk Institute for Biological Studies in California, researchers compared mice fed the same amount of high-fat food around the clock, to those fed over a period of eight hours.[9] They discovered that the mice who ate around the clock were more prone to obesity, high cholesterol and high blood glucose; while the mice given a restricted time in which to eat, weighed 28 per cent less and showed no adverse health effects, despite ingesting the same number of calories from the same fatty food. They also suffered less liver damage and systemic inflammation.

The findings have yet to be duplicated in humans, but according to the lead scientist Dr Satchidananda Panda, fasting overnight for 12 hours is potentially very beneficial for dieters and can 'override many of the negative effects of an unhealthy diet, including weight gain.'[10] This is because our metabolisms are programmed to expect a nightly fast. The digestive organs, particularly the liver, work at peak efficiency at certain times and 'rest' at others. During the day, the brain and muscles burn some of the calorific intake from carbohydrates for fuel, and the rest is stored in the muscles and liver in the form of glycogen. At night, the body converts the glycogen into glucose and releases it into the bloodstream to keep blood sugar levels steady while you sleep. Once the glycogen stores have been used up, the liver starts burning fat cells for energy. But if you are topping up your calorific intake late at night, or during those 'resting' hours, then the liver will not have a chance to go into fat-burning mode.

The conventional medical establishment will tell you that a calorie is a calorie, no matter what time of day it is eaten. And certainly, it is true that if you overeat wildly during the day, fasting for 12 hours at night will not have a magical slimming effect. But preliminary research suggests that giving your body a temporary break from food digestion helps to maintain insulin sensitivity, which makes it less likely that glucose will be stored as fat.[11]

Practitioners of Ayurvedic medicine meanwhile, have long advised eating lightly in the evening and no later than 6.00 pm, in addition to going for a walk after dinner, as going to bed with a full stomach can cause sleep disturbances and lead to lethargy in the morning.

It also helps to go to bed early, since night owls consume an average of 248 calories more per day and are heavier than those who go to bed earlier, according to a study at Northwestern University in Chicago in 2011.[12] Researchers found that those who go to bed late and sleep late, also eat more fast food, and fewer fruits and vegetables.

3. Soup for dinner is the dieter's best friend

Numerous studies have shown that soup aids weight loss and for this reason, it plays a key role in the Marie Antoinette Diet. Firstly, eating soup before a meal acts as an appetite suppressant by making you feel fuller sooner, so that you eat less for your main course. In a study by Dr Barbara Rolls and Julie Flood, at Pennsylvania State University, published in *Appetite* in 2007, 60 participants who ate soup as a first course reduced their total calorie intake at a given meal by

20 per cent, compared with those who did not have soup beforehand.[13]

In a prior study at Pennsylvania State University in 1999, Dr Rolls and her colleague Elizabeth Bell gave 24 women a 270-calorie starter of chicken-rice casserole, firstly on its own, secondly with a glass of water and thirdly by blending the casserole with the glass of water and serving it as soup.[14] Although the starters amounted to the same ingredients, when the participants ate them as soup they ate a third less calories for their main course, compared to when they ate the casserole alone or the casserole accompanied by a glass of water. The conclusion: when water is blended with food, the effect is more filling.

Using ultrasound and MRI scans scientists have researched what happens in the stomach after eating solid food taken with a separate glass of water at meals, compared with the same ingredients made into soup.[15] It seems that when you eat food, a valve at the bottom of the stomach, called the pyloric sphincter, holds food back until the digestive juices have had a chance to do their work. But when you drink water, the sphincter allows it to pass straight through to the intestines. This means that water that is drunk with food does not contribute to satiation or the feeling of being full. The scans confirmed that when the same ingredients are eaten as a soup however, the entire mixture remains in the stomach for digestion – and the stomach stays fuller for longer – because the water and food are blended together.

Satiety, the feeling of being full, is the new buzzword in dieting because when the stomach is empty, cells in the stomach wall release a hormone called ghrelin. Discovered by US scientists in 1999, ghrelin is thought to be key to hunger control, since it is carried via the bloodstream to the hypothalamus, the brain's appetite centre, to announce that it's time to eat.[16] (Previous studies have shown that when rats have ghrelin injected into their bloodstreams, they feed voraciously and become obese.)

Decreasing ghrelin levels could therefore be the key to combating obesity. Since soup fills up the stomach for longer, it effectively depresses this ghrelin activity and inhibits the switching on of the hunger signal.

Soup has been described as 'a miracle in a bowl for fat loss' for other reasons too. It is a good way to boost your liquid intake and stay hydrated; it is easy to digest; and it can deliver a significant dose of vitamins and minerals, since vegetables cooked directly in soups conserve more of their nutrients than those that are fried or boiled (and the water thrown away). In addition, soups, especially those with added pulses such as lentils or cannellini beans, can be a good source of fibre, which not only contributes to the feeling of satiety but also helps to balance blood sugar by slowing down the absorption of food.

Those who've tried the infamous Cabbage Soup Diet – based on eating as much cabbage soup as you want for seven days and created by doctors to lower the weight of dangerously obese patients prior to surgery – will know that it acts as a kind of internal colonic irrigation, sweeping all before it. Cabbage has many diet-friendly properties, but eating a diverse range of soups helps to prevent diet boredom and is an easy way to increase your intake of a wide selection of vegetables and other nutritious ingredients.

And although it is not borne out by science, alternative health practitioners believe that certain soups can address specific ailments as well as supporting key organs such as the kidneys and liver, and the adrenal glands (more of which later). For all these reasons, soup, either before a meal or as a replacement for it, really is the dieter's best friend.

4. The 18th-century diet had many advantages over the modern diet (and was less likely to lead to weight gain)

Some experts believe that to avoid modern day 'plagues' such as obesity, cancer and diabetes, we should eat the same foods as our far-off ancestors consumed. Advocates of the Paleolithic Diet for example, recommend a regime based on the diet of the Stone Age – fish, grass-fed meats, eggs, vegetables, fruit and nuts – and believe that we should eat similar food, because genetically, the human body has not changed much since then.

But this overlooks the fact that lifestyles have. Many people lead a sedentary existence and few of us are required to run around with a spear for several days in pursuit of lunch, or endure an enforced fast until the next 'kill' comes along. And as sceptics point out, we cannot be sure what our ancestors ate in the Stone Age; we can only guess. (And since one guess is raw bison intestines, containing half-digested seeds and grasses, I'm personally not rushing to revisit the cave-dwelling era.)

We do however, know what they ate in 18th-century France, thanks to the cookbooks of the time. Marie Antoinette's diet would have been based on meat, dairy, vegetables and fruit – what Dr Catherine Shanahan MD calls 'authentic' cuisine, as opposed to the factory-processed. In her book, *Deep Nutrition: Why Your Genes Need Traditional Food*, Dr Shanahan identifies 'four pillars' of 'authentic cuisine', which include meat cooked on the bone, organ meats (liver, kidneys and other offal), and fresh vegetable and animal products such as milk.

We can all benefit from eating the diet of an era when hydrogenated fats did not exist and food did not come wrapped in plastic. There is no doubt that real food – and by this I mean eggs, butter, cheese, whole milk, meat from organic, ideally grass-fed animals and soups based on homemade stock (more of which later) – is healthier and more conducive to weight loss than foods featuring unnatural ingredients and additives. But is it necessary to return to the Stone Age to find this 'authentic cuisine'? The more I read about the 18th-century diet – at least that of the reasonably affluent, since the poor lived mostly on bread and soup – the more I became convinced of its benefits and nutritional superiority to the modern diet.

I'm not suggesting that we revert to eating dishes such as songbird ragout or calves' hooves in whipped cream, but rather a return to ingredients and culinary techniques that have endured across many cultures through the ages – or foods 'culled from the centuries, the cream skimmed off the milk of time', as the American physician, Dr Henry Bieler, author of *Food Is Your Best Medicine*, wrote of his diet-based remedies in 1965. Many of the signature dishes in the contemporary French diet actually date back to the 18th century and beyond – dishes that have proven their nutritional worth for many generations. The desserts featured in Menon's *La Cuisinière Bourgeoise* (*The French Family Cookbook*) published in 1746, for example, are the same desserts that dominate the menu in French restaurants today – namely fruit tarts and custard-based puddings such as *œufs à la neige* ('eggs in snow') and crème caramel.

The food of Marie Antoinette's era would have naturally contained more nutrients than the modern-day equivalent, because a higher proportion of livestock would have been fed on pasture and raised in sunlight rather than in industrial sheds. By the end of the 18th century, forward-thinking physicians such as George Cheyne and the philosopher Jean-Jacques Rousseau had worked out basic principles of nutrition that seem even more relevant today. Cheyne for example, opposed the intensive farming of cattle and poultry. He believed that confining animals to stalls or barns and fattening them up unnaturally, made such animals unfit sources of food. 'Perpetual foulness and cramming, gross

39

food and nastiness, we know, will putrefy the juices and mortify the muscular substance of human creatures; and ... thus make even our food poison ... The only way of having sound and healthful animal food is to leave them to their own natural liberty, in the free air... with plenty of food and due cleanness,' he wrote.[17] Both Cheyne and Rousseau also questioned the nutritional value of vegetables and fruits grown out of season in hot beds; while Cheyne believed that boiling and roasting were the healthiest cooking techniques, as frying added fatty particles that could cause bodily 'obstructions'.

Our 18th-century ancestors had much closer links to the food chain than most of us do today. Not only would they have known their suppliers, many would have grown or reared their food, themselves. In France, some of those links have been maintained: many people prefer to buy at the local baker, butcher and *traiteur* (delicatessen) and the people in my village still shop for fish, fruit and vegetables and cheeses in the local market, quizzing suppliers about their production methods before buying. This direct contact with suppliers is not so common in the UK, where the majority of people only shop in supermarkets, buying dry, packaged food and ready-meals containing meat that might well have done a tour of Europe before landing in their fridge. What has all this got to do with losing weight you might ask? Well, keep reading.

Homemade versus industrial food

Much modern food is over-processed and lacking in nutrients, giving rise to 'over-fed and undernourished syndrome', whereby even severely overweight people are lacking in nutrients because they've been eating poor quality food. Ready-meals, packaged baked goods and processed carbohydrates offer little in the way of nutrition, while dumping a lot of rubbish in your body. Avoiding commercially processed food is therefore one of the very best things you can do for both your health and for weight loss. As the singer Boy George recently said of his dramatic weight loss, 'The rule is, if it's got an advert, don't eat it.' Processed food rarely leaves you satiated. Instead, the spike and subsequent crash in blood sugar, makes you crave more, which is exactly what the manufacturers want.

Research in the US has shown that high-sugar processed foods can be as addictive as cocaine and nicotine in human beings, hijacking the brain in a similar way and overriding human will and judgment.[18] (There are even similarities in the language of food and drug addiction, with the term 'chocoholic' for example, used to describe people who cannot resist chocolate.) Using brain scans, researchers at Brookhaven Institute in the US, found that if obese people are shown pictures of their favourite foods, an area of the brain responsible for decisions experiences a surge of the feel-good chemical dopamine.[19] Cocaine addicts undergo a similar reaction when shown a bag of white powder.

Some food manufacturers manipulate this sugar-addiction in order to increase sales. The food industry has even coined a phrase, the 'bliss point',[20] to describe the precise amount of sugar, fat and salt required to produce ecstasy in the taste buds, and hook the consumer on its products. There is a reason why it is difficult to eat just one cookie from the packet. Conversely, when you start to put nutritious, quality food into your body, the less you crave junk, and the easier it becomes to walk past the quick-fix foods in the supermarket.

In some cases food production appears to have become a dark art with multi-national companies driven to using the cheapest ingredients that they can get away with. And, as the 2013 horsemeat scandal in Europe demonstrated, we have no idea what is going into some ready-meals and manufactured food. The only way to control what you are putting into your body, and ultimately your weight, is to cook it yourself. Sadly, many people claim that they are too busy. It's striking that the current tsunami of obesity coincides with a decline in the number of meals cooked at home. A 2011 survey in the UK by kitchen appliance maker Kenwood[21] revealed that only one in four meals in Britain is now home-cooked from scratch – a 30 per cent drop since the 1980s. Another UK survey of 2000 parents by the Department of Health revealed that 71 per cent are too busy to cook, while 96 per cent admitted feeding their family ready-made meals.[22] Only 16 per cent of those surveyed, cooked a meal from scratch every day; and a mere 90 people out of the 2000 surveyed said they never used convenience foods to prepare meals. It doesn't take a team of scientists to suggest there might be a link between the decline in home-cooked meals and the threefold increase in UK obesity levels since the 1980s.[23]

The proliferation of coffee bars and sandwich chains meanwhile, has led to an increasing number of people eating fast food for lunch – with all the processed vegetable oils, sugar and additives which that implies. There are many studies demonstrating that the more meals that are eaten away from home, the higher the risk of weight gain and obesity. A 2007 survey for example, found that individuals who consumed at least 25 per cent of their daily calories from foods and beverages away from their home were more likely to have a greater daily calorie intake.[24] The analysis also included the type of restaurant – full-service or quick-service, with the latter most associated with weight gain. 'Our results suggest that the effect of food away from home consumed from quick-service restaurants is greater than the effect of [that] consumed from full-service restaurants on body mass index,' the researchers concluded.

The soaring obesity rate in the UK goes hand in hand with this explosion of the food-on-the-go culture. In at least two of the Western European countries where the obesity rate is lower than in the UK, the culture of either going home or visiting a full-service restaurant for lunch still prevails. In the French countryside, where I live, snack bars are almost non-existent and a three-course lunch is considered almost a sacred right.

Junk food doesn't just cause people to pile on the pounds. Several studies have linked consumption of junk food to depression, and brain disorders such as dementia, anxiety and mood swings. According to one study in Spain, participants who ate the most commercial and/or fast food were 51 per cent more likely to develop depression than those with the lowest rate of consumption.[25] The analysis of 8964 participants by scientists from the University of Las Palmas de Gran Canaria and the University of Granada, did not just take into account fast food (hamburgers, sausages and pizzas) but also commercial baked goods, including muffins, fairy cakes, doughnuts and croissants.

Junk food has also been shown to be a contributory factor in inflammation, an over-activity of the immune system, which has been linked to many illnesses including allergies, arthritis, asthma, diabetes, heart disease, hay fever, and periodontitis (gum disease). Trans fats, a common component of fast and manufactured food, are one of the main culprits. They have been associated with systematic inflammation[26] and higher body mass index as well as increased risk of heart disease.

5. Marie Antoinette did not eat trans fats, margarine or low-fat spreads

The 18th-century diet was free from artificial trans fats, which were still well over a century away from creation by food scientists. Made by a process called 'hydrogenation', whereby hydrogen is added to polyunsaturated fats, trans fats are now universally regarded as damaging to the human body, yet manufacturers continue to use them in baked goods and commercial frying because they are cheap and extend the shelf life of industrial food. Trans fats have been shown to interfere with insulin metabolism and enzyme systems in the body and to increase the risk of heart disease.[27] They have also been associated with weight gain.

In one six-year experiment, monkeys fed a diet high in trans fats showed a weight gain of 7.2 per cent, compared to a 1.8 per cent gain for those on a monounsaturated fat diet.[28] More research is needed to demonstrate that trans fats cause weight gain in humans, but such is the body of scientific evidence against trans fats that they are banned in several countries. Denmark introduced laws strictly regulating the sale of many foods containing trans fats in March 2003, effectively removing partially hydrogenated oils from food for human consumption; while Switzerland banned trans fats in 2008.[29] In the US, California became the first *state* to ban them in restaurants starting in 2010; and in 2008, New York was the first *city* to outlaw trans fat use in restaurants – both in frying and in margarines and spreads – although (at the time of writing) the ban does not extend to packaged foods.

Sadly, Britain – with the exception of the high street chain Marks & Spencer, which has eradicated trans fats from its own-label food ranges – lags woefully behind, as does France. Supermarket shelves in both these countries still contain foods that include hydrogenated and partially hydrogenated oils, while some restaurants and fast food outlets continue to use trans fats and partially hydrogenated vegetable oils for frying, which in my opinion, is nothing short of scandalous. The single most important thing that governments could do to halt the spread of obesity and improve public health is to ban these fats, which have been described as akin to putting 'melted Tupperware' into your body, but the ministers responsible refuse to act, possibly for fear of upsetting the food industry.

Marie Antoinette by contrast, ate freshly churned butter, milk and cream – exactly the kind of food that we are advised to avoid if trying to lose weight. For over forty years, saturated animal fats have been regarded as public enemy number one for heart health and weight loss. But Dr Mary Enig, the respected biochemist and nutritionist, now retired but known around the world for her research into fats and oils – she was one of the first to warn against the dangers of trans fats – has long argued that the opposite is true. The medical profession and food manufacturers, she says, have dangerously misled the public over fats. For years, she points out, various government agencies and medical organizations in the US, including the American Heart Association, encouraged people to replace traditional saturated fats with partially hydrogenated oils in order to reduce the risk of heart disease – advice which seems laughable now, given what we know about trans fats and their artery-clogging effects.

But according to Dr Enig, it is not just hydrogenated and trans fats that we should worry about. Manufactured vegetable oils, including sunflower and corn oils, she says are unnatural, more likely to lead to weight gain and more damaging to the human body than animal fats. When heated to high temperatures and subjected to toxic extraction processes, the polyunsaturated fats in some vegetable oils, which are still promoted as healthy fats by the medical profession, are unstable and difficult for the body to process. 'Unpaired electrons located at the double bonds make these oils highly reactive,' says Dr Enig.[30] 'When they are subjected to heat or oxygen, as in extraction, processing, and cooking, free radicals are formed. It is these free radicals, not saturated fats, which can initiate cancer and heart disease. As such, industrially processed polyunsaturated oils, such as corn, safflower, soy and sunflower oils, should be strictly avoided.' Saturated fats, including butter, lard and goose fat on the other hand, are highly stable and less likely to form dangerous free radicals when heated.

That's not the only conventional wisdom that Dr Enig turns on its head. In *Eat Fat, Lose Fat: The Healthy Alternative to Trans Fats*, the influential book that she co-wrote with Sally Fallon, food industry researcher and co-founder of the Weston A Price Foundation (a non-profit organization in America, which aims to promote good nutrition), the authors argue that the best way to lose fat is to eat fat. Natural saturated fats, they claim, will boost your energy, improve digestion and increase your overall health and wellbeing; while the widely accepted belief that saturated fats cause heart disease, is a myth.

There are, of course, many studies supporting the conventional medical wisdom that high-cholesterol and saturated fats do promote heart disease. But certain scientists and medics believe that several key studies, linking dietary intake of cholesterol and saturated fats to cardiovascular disease, are flawed and that the association might not be as strong as has been previously suggested. Some of the research has focused on dietary intake of saturated fats, for example, without assessing other, potentially more significant, factors such as overall body fat or sugar intake.

Meanwhile, other studies completely contradict the received wisdom that saturated and animal fats should be avoided. A Yale University study in 2005 explored the effect of egg consumption on the inner lining of blood vessels.[31] In the study, 49 healthy adults were assigned to eat two eggs daily for six weeks. The experiment showed that this had no effect on total cholesterol and did not adversely affect the blood vessels, thereby supporting the view that 'dietary cholesterol may be less detrimental to cardiovascular health than previously thought'. Even more interesting was a second Yale study in 2010, examining the effect of daily egg consumption on 40 adults with high cholesterol rather than normal cholesterol.[32] Once again, the researchers found that the cholesterol from consuming two eggs a day for six weeks was not detrimental to the participants' cholesterol levels or the functioning of the linings of blood, heart and lymphatic vessels.

Another study in 2012 suggests that one type of saturated fat, known as stearic acid – found in beef and pork, skinless chicken, olive oil, cheese, chocolate and milk – may actually protect against heart disease.[33] The research revealed that eating lean beef on a daily basis improved cholesterol levels. After five weeks on the diet of daily lean beef, participants in the study experienced a 5 per cent drop in total cholesterol and around a 4 per cent drop in 'bad' LDL cholesterol. This positive change was attributed to the stearic acid in the meat. Dr Michael Roussell, one of the study authors from Pennsylvania State University, said that, unlike processed meats such as sausages and ham, unadulterated red meat 'brings a unique, heart-healthy blend of fats to the table'.[34]

The authors of *Eat Fat, Lose Fat* meanwhile, make the further claim that high cholesterol does not lead to heart disease, pointing out that cholesterol is needed of many bodily functions, including protection against free radical damage, the repair of damaged cells and mineral metabolism. They cite several studies that suggest it is low cholesterol rather than high cholesterol that is the problem. A 1989 analysis[35] of elderly women published in *The Lancet* for example, found that the women who lived the longest were those with very high serum cholesterol (the total cholesterol level in a person's blood, both 'good' and 'bad'). Women with very low serum cholesterol levels had a death rate over five times higher.

But because of the accepted belief that cholesterol-rich foods are dangerous, we have over the past few decades, been encouraged to reduce or remove many nutrient and vitamin-rich foods like eggs, cream, butter and liver, from our diet, or wherever possible, replace them with low-fat versions. Yet many nutrition experts believe that natural foods are better for the body than those that have been synthetically engineered. Low-fat and no-fat foods, they argue, are another food industry sham, as they contain high concentrations of sugar to compensate for the reduced fat. In the body, excess sugar is converted into fat, so you might as well eat the natural full-fat version in the first place. Personally, I'd rather have real butter – Marie Antoinette is said to have churned her own while playing at her favourite pastime of being a milkmaid – and eat less of it.

As you might have guessed, I'm firmly in the pro-saturated fat camp and with the exception of olive oil, I avoid vegetable oils that have been industrially processed. However, I should add a couple of notes of caution. Firstly, butter and cream are high in calories, so if you are trying to lose weight, it's a good idea to limit intake for that reason. Secondly, although the research is contradictory, as already stated, many studies *have* shown that an excess of saturated fat can affect levels of 'bad' cholesterol in the body.

PART THREE

LOSING THE FIRST
FIVE KILOS – MY STORY

When I mentioned Marie Antoinette's eating habits to my French female friends, they nodded knowingly, as if dinner of soup and a 'wing of fowl' was no big news to them. I felt as if I was finally being admitted to the sisterhood of the svelte *Française*. I'd been eating French food but had gained weight, as I wasn't eating it the French way.

French women rarely discuss diets and never admit to being on one. Calorie control, for them, is a very private affair. But by further probing my friends' eating habits, I discovered one of the real reasons why French women stay slim: like Marie Antoinette, many of them eat very lightly in the evening. They also secretly juggle or balance out their calories on a daily basis. French women do not flinch when a slab of fatty terrine or a crème caramel is placed before them at lunchtime, because they know that they will redress the balance by eating lightly at dinner, and vice versa: if they are going out for dinner, they rein themselves in at lunchtime or the next day. Then, when I started to question my French friends in more detail, they admitted that their dinner often consisted of little more than a bowl of soup with a salad and a piece of cheese. (Tellingly, the old French word for a light evening meal is *le souper*, from which the English word 'supper' is derived.)

Unlike the French queen, I had grown accustomed to imbibing most of my calories late at night. After taking the dog for his evening walk, I'd pour myself a glass of wine (a ritual that I'd picked up in the three years that I lived with a French boyfriend) and start to prepare an elaborate evening meal such as boeuf bourguignon, coq au vin or venison stew – the sort of rich dishes that the French traditionally eat at lunchtime. I was in France. I certainly hadn't come here to eat cheese on toast for dinner. But because these dishes take several hours to prepare, I would often eat as late as 10.00 pm, and then wonder why I woke up the next morning feeling as if I'd run a marathon.

Tired (literally) of this situation, I decided to make some changes. Breakfast, I decided, would remain the same: half a sliced apple with a plain, full-fat yoghurt topped with a few chopped pecans or walnuts, followed by a coffee and a pain au chocolat. Although I can hear the tut-tutting of nutritionists, the latter was non-negotiable since I relied on the combination of sugar, carbohydrate and caffeine to kick-start my brain in the morning. But I decided to make one significant change: I would eat my main meal at lunchtime, which instinctively felt like a healthier thing to do. A glance at world obesity statistics, meanwhile, proved interesting. In the US and the UK, two of the countries with the biggest obesity problem, most people take in most of their calories in the evening. Strangely, there is very little scientific analysis of how timing of the main meal affects obesity. But it struck me as significant that countries where people traditionally eat their largest meal at lunchtime, such as Sweden and Spain, rank much lower in the obesity charts. (In Spain, on average, 40 per cent of the daily calories are taken at lunch.[36])

As serendipity would have it, my lifestyle overhaul coincided with the reopening of the café in my village and the arrival of a new chef offering a three-course daily lunch for €12. The menu was entirely homemade – nothing from industrial catering cans – and it was varied: gazpacho soup and steak with green beans, followed by pear charlotte, one day; squash soup, chicken and vegetables, and white chocolate mousse, on another. As an experiment, I decided that for one week I would join the locals, including the village doctor, the vet and a local farmer, for lunch in the café. Then in the evening, I would make like Marie Antoinette and eat soup and a salad.

The soup I decided, had to be homemade, using fresh ingredients, as would have been the case with Marie Antoinette's broth. (At Versailles, the *Potager du Roi,* or kitchen garden of the King, produced a wide array of fresh fruit and vegetables.) I had a small repertoire of soups that I could make without recourse to a recipe book and I started with those: carrot and coriander; watercress; and cabbage soup. I figured that I would have more than one bowl if I was hungry, but I wouldn't eat a thing after 8.00 pm. The results were apparent in a few days. After just two evenings of having soup and a salad for dinner, my stomach had noticeably shrunk. By day three, my stomach, while still far from flat, was moving in that direction and I'd lost a kilo. Within a week I had lost 2 kilos and suddenly I couldn't wait to get up in the morning and jump on the scales.

In the second week, I continued with my soup-for-dinner regime but I made lunch at home, rather than eating out. While I tried to keep it healthy and low GI, avoiding large helpings of carbohydrate, I pretty much ate what I wanted. But I made a point of not eating any manufactured food. Lunch continued to be the main calorie event of the day – often I prepared it the night before so that I wouldn't deviate from my regime – and I started to pay more attention to portion size.

My week of lunching in the local restaurant had proved enlightening. Although the French are perceived to eat huge amounts of food in those multi-course lunches that they are so fond of, the reality is that the sum of those courses adds up to a relatively small amount of food. And yet, because of the variety of foods you are eating, and because the meals are usually well balanced, you always feel full.

I tried to incorporate these principles at home. Rather than eat a big plate of pasta for lunch, I would eat a small bowl of pasta with a homemade sauce and accompany it with a brightly-coloured salad, consisting of at least five different vegetables – typically lettuce or watercress leaves, shredded carrot and red cabbage, half an avocado, tomatoes and bean sprouts – so that the bowl of pasta became almost the side dish and the salad the main event.

Another small but significant change was to swap my large white porcelain plates for a small cereal bowl, which led to an automatic adjustment in portion size. It's astonishing how much less you eat when serving food in a small bowl, which is possibly one of the reasons why the Japanese stay so slim. With the exception of bread, which I buy from the local bakery, everything I ate was homemade; while dinner was always soup and a salad, sometimes with a small chicken leg or thigh. And almost without noticing it, I cut out wine with dinner. This proved surprisingly easy, as a glass of Bordeaux doesn't lend itself quite so well to soup and a salad as it does to rich, highly flavoured food.

After fourteen days on my bespoke regime, I had lost just over 3 kilos (6.6lb), which is slightly over the recommended rate of weight loss of ½ to 1 kilo (1–2lb) a week. (Weight loss that is initially high can be due to fluid fluctuations rather than fat loss, so slow and steady is the way to go if you want to keep it off.) Eating lightly in the evening, I discovered, has other benefits too: namely, that I slept more soundly and instead of greeting the day like a drugged slug, I woke up with a clear head, feeling energized. Suddenly, I felt like a mistress of the universe and had enough energy for a morning run around the local lake with the dog. I cooked in advance and froze the soups, so that I was never tempted to pour myself a glass of wine and eat crisps while waiting for dinner to cook.

In the third week of my diet, I introduced a couple of other changes. Firstly, I replaced my daily pain au chocolat with a slice of homemade cherry and almond cake (see p. 158), which had a similar amount of calories – 215 calories in a 50g (just under 2oz) portion – but was more filling and nutritious. At the same time, I gradually reduced the sugar in my coffee from one teaspoon to none, having read that drinking your sugar – be it in tea, coffee, fruit juice, sports or fizzy drinks – is one of the worst things that you can do for weight gain, as it causes blood glucose levels to soar. (Marie Antoinette's habit of adding sugary syrup to her drinking water is a practice that I don't recommend adopting on this diet. Ditto her daily bowl of thick hot chocolate.) A year ago, the thought of drinking coffee without sugar would have been unthinkable to me, but if you have cake with your morning shot of caffeine, you really don't need sugar too. The bitter taste of Arabica beans actually serves as a counterpoint to the sweetness of the cake.

By the end of the third week, I'd lost another kilo, making a total of 4 kilos (8.8lb). The amazing thing was that I never really felt as though I was on a diet. One Saturday afternoon, cupboards cleared of the usual chocolate bars and biscuits in order to avoid temptation, I whipped up pancakes to kill a sugar craving. Served with fresh lemon juice and a dash of maple syrup, they took less than five minutes to make and, unlike industrial snacks which seem to make you hungry for more, one was enough.

In the fourth week, I did not stick to my diet so rigidly, as I had planned several evenings out with friends. But if I was at home, I continued to have soup and salad for dinner and I also took the dog for a longer walk the following day, in order to maintain the weight loss. Despite eating two full-blown restaurant dinners with wine and dessert, that week, I lost another kilo, making a total of 5 kilos (11lb) in four weeks. I was half way to my target weight loss. I can't say that it was all plain sailing as there were some evenings when I did go to bed feeling very hungry; and once or twice I cheated. But when I found myself eating a single square of dark chocolate late one evening, and savouring every nibble, I felt as if I'd finally morphed into a French woman, since prior to the diet, scarfing down an entire bar of cheap milk chocolate would have been much more my style. (Incidentally, not only is dark chocolate healthier but science has demonstrated that it is more filling than milk chocolate and reduces cravings for sweet, salty and fatty foods.[37])

Eager to expand my culinary repertoire beyond the cabbage and watercress soups that I'd been dining on and stave off diet boredom, I started experimenting with different recipes, looking at the nutritional benefits of various ingredients and specific foods that can help with weight loss. It was while doing this research, that I stumbled upon a very interesting discovery – a centuries-old recipe for a soup with supposedly astonishing health benefits, but relatively unknown in the western world: bone broth.

Made from boiling the bony and cartilaginous parts of the chicken (or lamb or beef), this broth is considered by its advocates, of which there are many, to boast a multitude of healing properties. In traditional Chinese medicine, it is believed to be a powerful medicine for the kidneys and adrenal glands. It is also said to promote strong teeth and bones, the kidneys and bones being related in Chinese medical theory. I became very excited when I realized that bone broth was almost certainly the broth that Marie Antoinette would have eaten every night at Versailles. It subsequently became the basis of my weight loss plan. In the next section, I'll explain in greater detail how the Marie Antoinette Diet works in practice.

PART FOUR

THE PRACTICE

1. You can eat cake but do so early in the day

For me, a day without coffee and cake is a day not worth getting out of bed for. I decided early on, that my bespoke regime would have to factor in those weaknesses. Cake is therefore allowed on the Marie Antoinette Diet, so long as you follow a few simple rules.

The first is that you start the day with a healthy breakfast. This means fruit – berries in summer; half a chopped apple or pear in winter – with yoghurt and a teaspoon of chopped pecans or walnuts sprinkled on top. Assuming that the portion of fruit weighs 80g (2.8oz), this ticks off one of the five-a-day fruit and veg requirement early on, starting the day with points in the nutritional bank, while the berries provide a perky dose of vitamin C.

You can follow this with coffee and cake, either immediately or an hour or so later. The Marie Antoinette Diet was not designed to be overly prescriptive or involve calorie counting, but it does require you to exercise commonsense with regards to portion size. For the avoidance of doubt, that means your slice of cake should be a maximum of 75g (2.6oz). To give you some idea, a fresh cream chocolate éclair which is my particular weakness, weighs around 75g. Some might find it odd that I have included cake in a weight-loss regime, but it's my belief that banning sweet things can cause cravings that ultimately lead to you ditching the diet. Yes, it's laudable and would be very beneficial to your health to try and eradicate sugar from your diet completely, but for most of us, the realistic alternative is to limit intake and to eat it in foods that also provide some nutrients.

There is, it has to be said, a growing body of evidence that sugar rather than fat is the culprit as far as the national free fall into obesity and diabetes is concerned. This is partly because manufacturers now routinely add it to foods that don't need it, such as bread, pizza and baked beans. Recently, I was shocked to find glucose syrup listed as an ingredient in organic stock cubes and even a can of crabmeat. It's true that we should all be eating less of the 'white poison', but that does not mean that you have to ban it altogether. Meals that contain sugar do not make the blood sugar rise any higher than meals that contain equal carbohydrate levels (pasta, bread or white rice, for example) but no sugar. The key factor is the glycemic load.

The glycemic index measures how quickly a fixed amount of carbohydrate raises glucose levels in the blood; but the glycemic load is a better indicator of how a food will affect blood sugar as it takes into account the quantity of carbohydrate, and therefore sugar, eaten.

In other words, as far as blood sugar management and obesity are concerned, sugar per se is not the problem; rather it is the *quantity* of it. Foods that contain too much sugar cause insulin to rise, which in turn makes it more likely that calories will be stored as fat cells. As with most things, the key is moderation, which is the mantra of many a svelte French woman.

Obviously, you'll lose weight faster if you forgo the daily pleasure of cake, and I feel duty-bound here, to flag up research showing that the caffeine and carb combo is very bad news for blood sugar levels and therefore for dieters. In a study at Canada's University of Guelph, participants were given a carbohydrate snack (in this case, a bowl of cereal) together with either a decaf or regular coffee.[38] Those on the caffeine and carb combo experienced a 250 per cent increase in blood sugar levels. At the same time, sensitivity to insulin, the hormone that controls blood sugar levels, was almost halved. This is a double whammy for dieters as high blood glucose levels and poor insulin function are both a recipe for weight gain and a diabetes risk, since the excess blood sugar is dumped as fat.

But even armed with this information, the morning fix of coffee and carbohydrate was non-negotiable for me as I rely on it to jolt my brain into gear. I know that nutritionists and doctors will not approve of that last statement, but to offset the indulgence, I try not to eat sugar after midday and if I have eaten cake for breakfast, I forgo dessert at lunch. I also keep the portion size small, so as not to create too much of a spike in blood sugar. And as part of my damage limitation, I take the dog out for a brisk walk immediately after my coffee and carb fix, as this helps to burn up the sudden surge of blood sugar.

2. If you are going to eat cake, bake it yourself (and only eat dessert if it's amazing)

Marie Antoinette, we know, ate cake and according to Madame Campan's memoirs, had a sweet tooth, but one thing is certain: the cake she ate did not contain any of the nasty ingredients that go into modern manufactured food. There are three main reasons why I recommend making cake rather than buying it. The first is that industrial sweets, biscuits and cakes usually contain a raft of bad-guy ingredients such as hydrogenated fats, monoglycerides and diglycerides (which may contain hidden trans fats) and other additives, which are added by manufacturers to either prolong shelf life or reduce production costs. By baking it yourself – and it is possible to make cake in batches, divide it into individual portions and freeze it in plastic bags or containers, which prevents you munching it all in one sitting – you can be certain that you are excluding these potentially harmful ingredients.

A second reason for making your own cake is that it is something of a reality check to see how much fat and sugar goes into a typical recipe. I recently made a chocolate cake by a well-known British chef and was so horrified by the giant slab of butter and pile of sugar that the recipe required, that the thought of eating the finished result made me feel quite nauseous. When you buy off-the-shelf baked goods, you are shielded from the reality of what you are eating. Reading the fat and sugar content as a statistic on the packaging does not have quite the same impact as seeing it in a menacing pile in the mixing bowl.

Thirdly, when making a cake yourself, you can adjust the sugar and fat content. As a general rule, you can reduce the stated sugar amount in most recipes by 20–30 per cent, usually without making any real difference to the taste.

Progressively cutting back the sugar in this way also helps to recalibrate your taste buds. Since I started baking my own cakes, the shop-bought versions now seem repellently sweet to me. By baking your own cakes, you can also play around with the recipe in other ways, substituting healthier ingredients such as oats for a proportion of the flour when making cookies, crumble toppings or cheesecake bases, for example. Wherever possible, I use flour made from spelt, an ancient form of wheat, for baking cakes, as it contains more protein and nutrients than ordinary wheat flour and has a lower glycemic index.

One ingredient that has become almost ubiquitous in industrial food production is glucose-fructose syrup or high-fructose corn syrup. It's increasingly difficult to find any manufactured products that do not contain this controversial liquefied sugar. High-fructose corn syrup is a man-made sweetener, invented in the mid-1960s and now used in many processed foods, including cakes, sweets, biscuits, ketchup, cereals, sodas and baked goods. Powerful food lobbies will vigorously deny that it is anything but safe, since chemically it is very similar to table sugar or sucrose, while some research has suggested that our bodies break down and use the two sweeteners in the same way.

However, many health experts believe that fructose syrup has no effect on satiety and aggravates insulin resistance. Numerous studies over the past few decades have provided cause for concern, showing that fructose syrup causes increased weight gain over other forms of sweeteners. In one study at Princeton University published in 2010,[39] rats that were fed high-fructose corn syrup gained fat 300 per cent more quickly than those fed an equal dose of table sugar, or sucrose. High-fructose corn syrup was also shown to augment visceral fat deposits around the belly – the most dangerous area to carry excess fat.

The theory is that, as a result of the manufacturing process, the fructose molecules in high-fructose corn syrup are free and unbound, and ready for absorption. By contrast, the fructose molecules in sucrose from cane or beet sugar are each bound to a corresponding glucose molecule and must undergo an additional metabolic step before they can be used or absorbed by the body. Professor Bart Hoebel, of the Princeton research team said, 'Some people have claimed that high-fructose corn syrup is no different than other sweeteners when it comes to weight gain and obesity, but our results make it clear that this just isn't true.'[40]

Another reason to dust down your baking tins is that cooking is an enjoyable process, associated with feelings of happiness. Whereas fast food is all about instant gratification, baking a cake is a deferred pleasure. A kitchen filled with the wonderful scent of vanilla, chocolate or ginger cooking, is a slowly unfurling treat for the senses, and ultimately more pleasurable than unwrapping a quick industrial sugar fix. The principle of delayed gratification, incidentally, is a cornerstone of the French approach to food. One reason why French women do not snack between meals is that it lessens the pleasure of the next lunch or dinner.

For all these reasons, eating cake or dessert that is homemade, from scratch – and that means no shortcuts with ready-made pastry, toppings or fillings – is one of the basic tenets of the Marie Antoinette Diet. And if you're serious about your health and losing weight, the general principle, 'If it's industrial, don't eat it', should also apply in restaurants, especially with regards to desserts.

The first thing I do when the waiter brings the dessert menu in France is to ask him to point out the dishes that are *fait maison* or homemade. If the chef has made the dish himself from scratch, fine, but if it has been bought as a job lot from an industrial supplier, then it's a mass-produced pleasure that I'm happy to forgo. So the rule I follow is,

'Only eat dessert if it's amazing.' And if it's from a factory, it probably isn't.

Tips

- Look for dessert recipes that include nuts such as almonds, walnuts or pecans, for extra nutritional benefits.
- Always check labels and avoid food and drinks containing high-fructose corn syrup.
- When making cakes, add the sugar gradually to the mix, and keep tasting the batter until you reach an acceptable level of sweetness.
- Substitute oats for a proportion of the flour wherever appropriate – when making cookies or crumble toppings, for example.
- Use spelt flour rather than wheat flour for baking cakes and biscuits, as it contains more protein and nutrients.
- Check food and drink labels and avoid products containing high-fructose corn syrup.
- Do not drink your sugar. Many sugared drinks and sodas now contain high-fructose corn syrup. Drinking them is one of the worst things you can do if you are trying to lose weight. Equally, by adding sugar to tea or coffee you are not only squandering calories and creating a

spike in blood glucose levels, but also sending fructose on a fast track to the liver where it will be metabolized into fat.

- If a cake recipe requires fat (usually butter), experiment by replacing up to half of the required amount with virgin coconut oil. Although butter is a good and very nutritious fat, many experts believe that coconut oil is the healthiest fat of all and the most rapidly burnt off by the body. I'll explain why, later.

Why Bake With Spelt?

The health benefits of spelt were recognized as far back as the Middle Ages when the Benedictine abbess, St. Hildegard von Bingen recommended it for many illnesses, proclaiming that 'Spelt creates a healthy body, good blood and a happy outlook on life.'

As well as containing more protein than flour made from typical wheat (15–21 per cent as opposed to around 9–13 per cent) it also contains more nutrients. It is a good source of the mineral manganese, which plays an important role in calcium absorption and blood sugar regulation, and also contains phosphorus, vitamin B3, magnesium and fibre.

Anecdotal evidence suggests that many people find spelt flour easier to digest than ordinary wheat flour, although the theory is not supported by science. Another advantage for dieters, is that bread made from spelt flour has a lower glycemic index than ordinary bread (with a GI of 54–60 as opposed to 61–73 for most wheat breads).

Although this ancient grain is in fact, a member of the wheat family – it was one of the first grains to be used for baking bread – it has a tougher outer shell, which makes it easier to grow with less recourse to pesticides. Unfortunately, the hard outer coating means that it is more difficult to mill and therefore more expensive.

Traditionally, spelt has been popular in Germany and Switzerland, but in the UK and France it has fallen out of fashion in recent decades and is now a speciality crop, although it looks set for a resurgence as more people discover its health benefits. At least one French farmer of my acquaintance who stopped growing spelt some time ago, is considering cultivating it again.

Spelt lends itself well to baking and has a pleasant nutty taste. But when using spelt flour for making cakes, you will need to add baking powder as it doesn't rise as much as the wheat equivalent. You might also find that you need to adjust the amount required. It depends on the product but I find that if a recipe calls for 175g of normal flour, it is likely to equate to 150g of spelt flour or less.

IMPORTANT NOTE: *Although some people with wheat intolerances find that their body can cope with spelt, it does contain gluten and is not suitable for diagnosed coeliacs.*

3. Eat your main meal at lunchtime and make it as low GI as possible

Of all the diets that I'd encountered before creating my own, there was only one that struck me as sensible and sustainable over the long term – the GI diet, based on the glycemic index (GI) of different foods. GI is the measure of how quickly a fixed quantity of a particular food is broken down by the body, and therefore, how rapidly it causes blood sugar to rise. By focusing on foods that break down slowly, thereby making you feel fuller for longer, the GI diet reduces the risk of diabetes and heart disease.

Marie Antoinette's diet would have been naturally low GI, as was 18th-century cuisine in general, relying as it did on meat, fish, vegetables and dairy products. So too, I've noticed, are the three-course lunch menus so widely offered by French restaurants. Slow-release foods such as lentils, green string beans and flageolet beans, which break down slowly and leave you fuller for longer, feature very strongly in French cuisine, while hunger-stoking carbohydrates such as potatoes, pasta and white rice are generally served in miniscule quantities, if at all.

The Marie Antoinette Diet allows you to eat pretty much whatever you want for most of the day, the exception being fried food in restaurants, for reasons that I will explain in more detail in the next section. It's also important to remember that when we eat carbohydrates like pasta, bread and cereals, the body metabolizes them as if they were sugar, promoting insulin production, an increase in blood sugar levels and the storage of fat. You can however, reduce the insulin spike by opting for carbohydrates with a lower GI such as seeded and granary breads, sweet potatoes and brown basmati rice.

Eating an early lunch, meanwhile, as is still the custom in much of rural France – in my local restaurant, you are pushing your luck if you ask for a table after 12.45 pm – might also be conducive to weight loss. A recent study in Spain[41] found that, of 420 people on a 20-week weight-loss programme, those who ate an early lunch, defined as before 3.00 pm for the Spaniards, lost 2.2kg (4.85lb) more than those who ate lunch later (9.9kg versus 7.7kg). Both groups ate the same number of calories: 40 per cent of their daily total was consumed at lunch, as is the custom in Spain, where lunch remains the main meal of the day. The study is regarded as inconclusive as it did not take into account other lifestyle factors, and more research is needed on how the timing of meals affects weight, but it does suggest a link between eating lunch early and weight loss.

Eating the bulk of your calories at lunchtime meanwhile, may have been the slimming secret of high profile French women through the ages. The Empress Josephine for example, unless she was dining with Bonaparte, would receive friends for lunch in her yellow salon at precisely 9.45 am.[42] And the meal, which was eaten at 11.00 am, would have been substantial, including soup, hors d'oeuvres, a roast, a series of side dishes or *entremets*, and sweets, followed by coffee and liqueurs.

Tips

- Make lunch your main meal of the day and eat it before 3.00 pm.
- Treat potatoes, rice, pasta and fries as if they are sugar — which is how they are perceived by the body — and only eat in small portions.
- Buy a small set of kitchen scales and get used to weighing

your carbohydrate before cooking it. Portions of pasta, rice or noodles should not exceed 50–75g (2–3oz) a serving, dry weight. This may seem like a small amount, but you do get used to it.

- Other than fries, there are no restrictions on what foods you can eat for lunch so long as you observe the following proportions: half your plate should be comprised of vegetables; one quarter, lean protein; and the remaining quarter, complex carbohydrates such as brown rice, sweet potatoes, quinoa, beans or lentils.

4. Eat soup for dinner

Soup for dinner, followed by a salad, is a cornerstone of the Marie Antoinette Diet. If you are really hungry you can accompany your salad, as the French queen did, with a small piece of chicken or, if you are vegetarian, cheese. One of the great advantages of soup is that it is a quick, filling and easy meal that can be prepared in advance. I make it up in large batches and freeze it in plastic containers, so that I always have at least half a dozen kinds to choose from and don't get bored.

The fact that the soup is pre-prepared is crucial to the diet's success. If you come home from work feeling tired and hungry, the chances are that you are not going to want to get busy with a chopping board and a blender – at least not, in my case, without reaching for a glass of wine and a handful of crisps first. The fact you have a nutritious dinner already made, means that you are less likely to resort to junk food. If you live alone, it actually feels quite liberating not to have to think about your evening meal. The other interesting thing about eating soup in the evening, I have noticed, is that it kills the craving for wine. I'm not sure why this is, but wine and soup just don't seem to mix.

You can, if you are really busy, buy ready-made soup, provided that it is not the canned variety, which usually contains a lot of salt, and that you check the label for undesirable additives, taste enhancers and sugar. (No one needs sugar in their soup, but it is surprising how many savoury foods now contain it.) Most supermarkets now sell freshly-made gourmet soups, which are free of additives, so if pressed for time, choose one of those. But generally, nothing beats a soup that you have made yourself. Some of the soup recipes that I've included at the end of this book can be rustled up in less than ten minutes. And, since soup is cheap to make and a good way to use any leftover vegetables lurking in your fridge, it is also a very economical way to eat.

If you do have a family to feed, it is a little more of a

challenge, but there is no reason why you cannot follow the soup regime and set aside a serving of the evening meal that you have cooked for your family, to have for your lunch the next day. This is what many French women do, making one meal stretch to two and taking the leftovers into the office to heat up for the following day's lunch.

Bone broth

When I first started my diet, I found myself wondering what went into Marie Antoinette's evening broth. One of the most popular cookery books of the era, *Le Cuisinier François*, written by François Pierre la Varenne in 1651, gives a typical recipe for bouillon: 'The way to make stock for the enrichment of all dishes, be it *potage* (soup), entrée or *entremet*,' he wrote, '[is to] get hind leg and rump of beef, a little mutton and a few fowl, depending upon the amount of the bouillon you want. Then cook it well with a bouquet and some cloves. Keep hot water at hand all the time to refill the pot. When it is done, strain it to make use of it.'

Hind leg. A few fowl. It's safe to say that more than a few bones were boiled in the making of Marie Antoinette's evening soup, and that it was almost certainly a bone broth. In the 18th century, it would have been quite normal to incorporate, among other things, chicken feet, necks, and offal such as liver, into a stock.

Although Marie Antoinette is unlikely to have been aware of it, she was eating a soup that has been advocated for centuries by practitioners of traditional Chinese medicine, who believe that bone broth nourishes the kidneys and supports the adrenal glands. Among the many other claims made for this magic soup are that it helps to heal damaged and swollen joints, gum disease and connective tissues, as well as strengthening bones and teeth and boosting the body's vital essence or *chi*. It is also said to promote youthful-looking skin. (It is perhaps not coincidence that Marie Antoinette was said by contemporary observers to have a glowing skin, while portraits of the Queen show her with a peaches and cream complexion.)

Many cultures around the globe have used bone broth for centuries as a healing tonic, particularly to alleviate joint problems and arthritis. This, devotees claim, is because it contains a series of proteins called glycosaminoglycans (GAGs for short), which make up collagen and support connective tissue throughout the body. In recent years, certain GAGs, namely glucosamine, chondroitin and hyaluronic acid, have been used as supplements to redress arthritis and support joint and skin tissues. But bone broth according to its proponents, is more effective than these synthesized preparations because it contains proteins in a more bioavailable form. As for the minerals, because they are naturally derived and extracted from bone, they are in an ideal balance and easily utilized by the body. The fats in the bone broth also facilitate the absorption of the minerals.

Advocates of bone broth also claim that it can help with adrenal fatigue, a syndrome denied by most conventional doctors but thought by others to be the reason for many common ailments, ranging from unexplained tiredness to autoimmune disorders, such as psoriasis and multiple sclerosis, which occur when the body's immune system mistakenly attacks its own tissues. Adrenal fatigue is also thought to be a contributory factor in adult-onset diabetes.

The adrenal glands are two small glands that sit above the kidneys and secrete cortisol and adrenaline, the hormones that help to deal with stress, as well as regulate blood glucose levels. The theory is that when forced to deal with years of stress, too many late nights, life events such as loss or bereavement, or over-reliance on stimulants such as sugar and caffeine, they become exhausted, leaving the sufferer worn-out, irritable, depressed and in the worst instances, unable to get out of bed for more than a few hours a day. Bone soup is said to help because it contains gelatin, which assists liver function and improves digestion, a process that otherwise uses up a lot of bodily energy.

The scientific evidence for bone broth?

So is there any scientific evidence to support these claims? The answer is that there has been very little research into bone broth other than a study carried out at King's College Hospital in London in 1934.[43] The researchers, Dr McCance and Dr Elsie Widdowson, respected names in the history of nutrition, examined the mineral salts released from veal bones when heated firstly alone, and then with vegetables (potatoes, onions, carrots and Savoy cabbage).

Although both broths contained magnesium, potassium, copper and phosphorus, the amounts were deemed too small to be significant. The scientific analysis did however, establish that the broth is alkaline in composition and contains as much calcium as a comparable size serving of milk. Despite this, the researchers concluded that, 'As judged by chemical standards, bone and vegetable broths are not of great nutritional value.'

The study did not however, evaluate the broth for tissue and bone-boosting glycosaminoglycans or GAGs. But by establishing that the broth contains significant quantities of calcium, the King's College research does support the theory that bone broth helps to strengthen the bones and reminer-alize the teeth, since calcium and phosphorus are the two main minerals of which teeth are made. The fact that the broth is alkaline rather than acid would also be beneficial.

The only other study of bone broth, published in 2011, examined the effect of concentrated bone broth on bone density in rabbits.[44] Mahmood Aljumaily at Mosul University in Iraq, found that the broth helped in the accel-eration of bone healing and that the bone density in rabbits had significantly increased by the end of the fifth week of dietary supplementation with bone broth, in comparison to a control group. 'The findings in this study support the common folk idea that this dietary supplementation enhances bone healing when given in the course of fracture healing for sufficient time,' Aljumaily concluded.

There have been no clinical studies of the effects of bone broth in humans, a fact that is no surprise to its proponents, who point out that most scientific research into nutrition is sponsored by food producers with profits to make. Who wants to fund research into boiled bones, they ask?

But research has been carried out into bone broth's close cousin, chicken soup, and several scientific studies have shown it to contain substances with a medicinal effect.

Using a recipe passed down by his wife's grandmother that included chicken, onions, sweet potato, parsnips, turnips, carrots, celery stems, and parsley, Stephen Rennard MD led a study at Nebraska Medical Center in the US, and concluded that chicken soup might have an anti-inflammatory activity on the body, useful for remedying symptoms of upper respiratory tract viral infections.[45] It was however, an in vitro, laboratory experiment, so further research on humans would be needed to establish the benefits conclusively.

Those who've found bone broth to be beneficial to their health, point out that bone broth has stood the test of time and been used as a health tonic in many cultures for centuries. Bone broth is especially important as a source of calcium in cultures that do not consume milk and cheese. For that reason, many people eat it on a daily basis in Asia.

The best kind of research, devotees argue, is to try the broth for a month or so and see how it makes you feel. That would be my recommendation too. Regardless of whether or not the various health claims have been scientifically proven, Marie Antoinette's broth does have significant nutritional benefits thanks, in part, to the added vegetables. It is also filling, low-calorie and delicious, which makes it the ideal one-pot dinner for dieters.

- Eat soup for dinner and fill up with a large, colourful salad or a bowl of steamed vegetables. Try a mix of watercress and salad leaves, chopped peppers, bean sprouts, chopped red cabbage, tomatoes and half an avocado, with a small serving (approximately a teaspoon) of feta cheese crumbled on top.
- Your evening salad should not include rice, potatoes or pasta, although it is fine to eat them at lunchtime in controlled quantities.
- Avoid commercial salad dressings. Instead, make your own coconut oil and balsamic dressing: one teaspoon of warm, melted coconut oil and a splash of balsamic vinegar.
- Alternatively, dress your salad with a squeeze of fresh lemon juice and a teaspoon of olive oil.
- Prepare soups in advance and freeze them.
- To boost the health benefits of soups, use bone broth rather than commercial stock cubes as the base.

5. Observe a 12-hour night fast

Fasting for 12 hours overnight is much more doable than a 24-hour fast, as you will be sleeping for most of it. If you can combine a 12-hour night fast with soup and salad for dinner for a week you should see significant weight loss – up to several pounds or a kilo in seven days – assuming that you are not gorging on doughnuts and chips the rest of the time. After that, the combination of soup for dinner and fasting for 12 hours, two nights a week, should keep the weight off. It means that you can go out for dinner with friends and eat normally, although preferably lightly in the evening, most of the time. That said, if I'm going out for dinner, I do try and rein it in at lunch that day in order to balance the books calorie-wise.

In past eras, and certainly in Marie Antoinette's time, eating early and observing a 12-hour overnight fast would have been a natural thing to do for the majority of the population, especially in winter, when people went to bed as soon as darkness fell, living *d'un soleil a l'autre*, (from one sun to the other). And pre-electricity in French rural areas, people went to bed when the sun went down in order to avoid spending money on candles. Modern life, by comparison, means that many of us are up at all hours, surfing the web and as a result, susceptible to midnight fridge raids.

The 12-hour fast also means refraining from alcohol during those hours. Although alcohol is not banned on this diet, it is best to avoid it even in the early evening, because it causes a blood sugar dip, which can propel you to the kitchen cupboard later.

IMPORTANT NOTE: *A night fast is not recommended for sufferers of diabetes or hypoglycemia, who need a bedtime snack to keep blood sugar levels steady through the night.*

Tips

- Avoid alcohol in the evening, as it will make it more difficult to observe the 12-hour overnight fast.
- If it is impossible to avoid eating late – because of a work function or if you are out with friends, for example – eat breakfast later the next day, so that you still observe a 12-hour fast.

6. Eat as little manufactured and processed food as possible

For reasons already described, it is important to avoid fast food and manufactured products in favour of the slow, traditional and home-cooked. In rural France eating a three-course lunch is not just for the idle rich, but a way of life for all sectors of the population. It usually means going home to dine – many workers have a two-hour break in the middle of the day – or going to a local restaurant.

Nearly all restaurants and cafés in France offer a set lunch menu at a reasonable price. In my village, you are as likely to see the village solicitor enjoying the €12 set menu, as local farmers, truck drivers and council workers. I appreciate that a three-course lunch is not practical or possible for most people – some of whom count themselves lucky if they are able to grab a sandwich at their desk – but with a little forethought the Marie Antoinette diet can easily be adapted.

A friend who works for a French company in the middle of the countryside, with no cafés or restaurants nearby, reports that her female colleagues bring in leftovers from the previous evening's meal and reheat them in the office microwave. They then follow their home-cooked main course with yoghurt, one of the French woman's key weapons against hunger, and a piece of fruit.

If you do not have access to a fridge and a microwave at work, and if it is not possible to eat lunch in a non fast-food restaurant – and I do appreciate that not everyone has access to cooked food of a reasonable price and quality, as is the norm in France – you can still adapt this diet. Even if you only follow it properly at weekends, and eat soup for dinner two or three nights during the week, you should still lose weight, albeit more slowly, particularly if you are observing the 12-hour fast and not scarfing snacks late at night.

Alternatively, if it's not possible to heat food at work or eat lunch in an appropriate restaurant, prepare a delicious salad for lunch with a piece of chicken, cold salmon or cheese, which you can follow with a homemade dessert; and then have soup and a plate of vegetables in the evening.

Tips

- Make your own frozen meals, by making extra portions of the meal you are cooking, and freezing them in individual containers. That way you will always have something in the freezer for lunch, or to take to work if you have access to a fridge and a microwave there.
- Make one meal into several. If you are roasting a chicken for example, keep back the carcass for soup, and some meat to turn into a stew or salad later in the week.

7. Eat the right fats – and, wherever possible, cook with coconut oil

Like many people, I thought I was doing my body a favour by using extra-virgin olive oil for frying and roasting vegetables. But when a health-conscious acquaintance was diagnosed with breast cancer and asked her consultant, a leading light in his field, for dietary advice, she was astonished that, in addition to recommending black cherries and watercress to help with her recovery, he strongly advised against cooking with virgin olive oil. This is because it has a lower smoke point than refined (non-virgin) olive oil, the 'smoke point' being the temperature at which an oil produces visible vapour and starts to degenerate.

Many health experts, I subsequently discovered, believe that virgin olive oil, along with vegetable oils such as corn, soy, safflower, sunflower and canola, should not be used for cooking. Research has shown that when certain vegetable oils are heated to normal frying temperatures, their molecular structure starts to break down, releasing toxic and potentially carcinogenic compounds called aldehydes.

In one Spanish study, researchers tested extra virgin olive, sunflower and virgin linseed oils, heating them to frying temperature in an industrial fryer for a period of 40 hours, which is roughly the length of time they would be used commercially in a restaurant.[46] When the cooked oils were analyzed, researchers found that the sunflower and flaxseed, both high in polyunsaturated fats (the supposedly 'healthy' kind recommended by the health establishment) had degraded significantly and created the most toxic aldehydes in the least amount of frying time.

The extra-virgin olive oil also generated aldehydes, which have been linked with neurological disorders and a variety of cancers, but to a lesser degree and after cooking much longer.

The Spanish study demonstrated that not only are these toxic chemicals ingested when food cooked in the oils is eaten, but they are also released into the air where they can be inhaled. These compounds are thought to interact adversely with proteins, hormones and enzymes in the body to impede its correct functioning and damage the lining of the arteries.

Saturated animal fats, including lard, butter and goose fat, on the other hand, are inert, so when heat is applied, there is a limit to the damage it can do. For this reason, many food and health experts recommend saturated fats over supposedly 'heart healthy' vegetable oils for cooking.

And there is one saturated fat that seems to ace all others in terms of possible benefits for health and weight loss – virgin coconut oil, the wonders of which, I first discovered at a naturopathic detox retreat in Spain. Coconut oil is the fat most easily utilized by the body because it contains medium-chain fatty acids (MCFAs) or triglycerides. These are smaller and more easily burned by the liver as energy, than the long-chain fatty acids found in vegetable oils, which are more likely to be stored as fat.

By providing a quick source of energy, coconut oil is thought to help with chronic fatigue. It also combats low blood sugar and supports the thyroid gland, as well as fighting pathogens in the digestive tract that contribute to fatigue. And its benefits don't stop there. According to Dr Mary Enig, coconut oil reduces levels of 'bad' cholesterol in the body and has an anti-viral and anti-bacterial effect. It also has strong anti-fungal qualities, helping to combat candida in the gut, for example. And because coconut oil has been shown to fire up the metabolism (and increase body temperature), it is also the key to the weight-loss diet outlined in *Eat Fat, Lose Fat*. In this book, the authors describe coconut oil as 'the queen of fats' and recommend eating a tablespoon of coconut oil 20 minutes before every meal – a total of three tablespoons a day – in order to stimulate weight loss.

Coconut oil is said to have a significant effect on satiation, so by eating a tablespoon before every meal, you will eat less calories because you will feel full more quickly. (Personally, I can't manage a tablespoon; I prefer to use a teaspoon of melted oil, along with a splash of balsamic vinegar, as a salad dressing.)

Until very recently coconut oil, which contains more saturated fat than butter, received a bad press – thanks largely to a study showing that when fed to animals, it increased cholesterol levels. However, the coconut oil used in the research was hydrogenated rather than the virgin, unprocessed, kind.

Coconut oil's reputation underwent a dramatic overhaul in 2007 when a clinical trial in Brazil, yielded surprising results.[47] Forty women with abdominal obesity, aged 20–40 years, were given daily dietary supplements consisting of either two tablespoons of coconut oil or two tablespoons of soybean oil over a 12-week period. They all followed a 'balanced' diet with the same number of calories and were told to walk for 50 minutes a day.

By the end of the study, both the soybean oil consumers and the coconut oil group had similar reductions in body mass index, but those consuming coconut oil saw a reduction in their waist measurements. Unprompted, members of the coconut oil group had also reduced their consumption of carbohydrates and increased their protein and fibre intake.

The researchers concluded that supplementing the diet with coconut oil 'seems to promote a reduction in abdominal obesity'. This was attributed to the fact that coconut oil is the most readily digested and utilized of all the saturated fats.

Like butter and other saturated animal fats, coconut oil has a stable composition and is less likely to decompose or turn rancid when heated. For all these reasons, I now use coconut oil for almost all cooking, not just for frying but also for baking cakes, substituting it for butter wherever appropriate. It's important to use virgin coconut oil as this means that it has not been exposed to high heat or chemicals in the extraction process. I use a cold-pressed, organic version by Lucy Bee, although there are other brands available. High-quality coconut oil is not cheap but it is an investment in good health – and on a daily basis, cheaper than a cappuccino from a coffee chain.

Tips

- Scrutinize labels and if a product contains hydrogenated fats, monoglycerides or diglycerides, step away. If it contains partially hydrogenated oils, sprint away.
- Avoid cooking with vegetable or seed oils. Instead, use saturated fats such as butter or coconut oil, which are more stable.

- Use raw, virgin coconut oil – in other words, additive-free and cold-pressed, which means it has not been subjected to high temperatures or chemicals.
- For a delicious and healthy salad dressing, combine a teaspoon of virgin coconut oil with 2–3 teaspoons of balsamic vinegar. (Coconut oil is solid at room temperature but you can melt it gently in a small dish by leaving it to stand in a bowl of hot water for a few minutes.)
- If you do cook with olive oil, avoid the virgin variety and choose a 'light' (refined) version, which will have a higher smoking point. If you live in the UK, Marks & Spencer and Waitrose both offer good lightweight olive oils. Non-virgin olive oils are usually thin and pale in colour, so look for oils that are more yellow than green.

8. Move for at least 20 minutes after eating

Marie Antoinette often liked to walk in the gardens of Versailles after dinner and it seems that she was on the right track here too. A US study at the Mayo Clinic in Rochester, Minnesota, in 2012, showed that walking or other light exercise after meals can reduce glucose levels by more than half in both healthy and diabetic people.[48] The researchers even suggested that substituting activities such as washing the dishes after a meal could have similar effects to walking.

This is because physical activity decreases the amount of glucose and fats that accumulate in the blood after eating, thereby stabilizing blood sugar levels and preventing the sugar from being laid down as fat. Physical activity within half an hour of eating also helps to rev up the metabolism, which burns energy and calories. By contrast, slumping on the sofa or sitting in front of a computer after dinner increases the chance of excess blood sugar being dumped as fat.

The study participants walked for 33.5 minutes after two of their daily meals. In general, it was found that walking began to affect glucose levels 10 minutes after the exercise started and the benefits extended until 5 minutes after it stopped. According to lead study author Yogish Kudva, MD, 'Minimal activity sustained for 30 minutes (walking 0.7 miles in 33 minutes) lowers post-meal glucose concentrations. Such activity has little or no risk for almost everybody.'

Tips

- The best thing you can do after eating, if you want to burn fat and reduce the risk of type 2 diabetes, is move.

- If you can't manage a walk, do 30 minutes of housework, even if it is only the washing up, instead.

9. Eat liver once a week

This might seem rather strange advice given that liver is high in cholesterol and currently so unfashionable that it has almost disappeared from the modern diet. Marie Antoinette is likely to have eaten it regularly, since in the 18th century, pounded liver was often used to enrich sauces and added to stock.

In her book, *Deep Nutrition: Why Your Genes Need Traditional Food*, Dr Catherine Shanahan advocates eating the 'nasty' bits of animals – the organs and offal – on the basis that they contain the biggest nutritional bounty. In the 18th century, offal-based dishes such as lambs' testicles, and gratin of stuffed calves' eyes[49] were considered delicacies. Nowadays many people find the idea of offal, or 'organ meat' as it is known in the US, quite repugnant. Even in France, where I have variously encountered, and eaten, pigs' trotters and ears, ox tails and tongues, head of veal and cow brains, cheeks and thyroid gland, it is rare to see liver on a restaurant menu.

Not only is it an acquired taste, some people find the idea particularly unappealing, as it is the organ that filters toxins and, therefore, part of the body's rubbish disposal system, although toxins are not actually stored in the liver, merely processed by them. The liver *is* however, the body's storehouse for nutrients, which means that it is packed with vitamins and minerals, making it, in my opinion, the most overlooked of 'superfoods'.

As I fine-tuned my diet, I started to buy liver once a week from an organic butcher, frying it along with some onions, in a sliver of coconut oil and serving it with brown basmati rice and green vegetables. The reason? I remembered a piece of advice given to me several years ago, by a leading nutritionist – namely, that a well-nourished body is less likely to succumb to cravings or addictions. This is a key principle if you are trying to lose weight. Vitamin and mineral deficiencies also affect your mood, and can make you tired, depressed and irritable. And since I wanted my diet to have the feel-good factor – no one wants to be lethargic or depressed while trying to lose weight – liver again seemed to be the answer, as it contains many of the nutrients needed to make you feel calm and happy, including folic acid, selenium and tryptophan, a pre-cursor of the feel-good hormone, serotonin.

A small weekly serving of liver is an excellent nutritional insurance policy if you are following a slimming regime. Liver is one of the best sources of vitamin A, iron and zinc, which among other functions, regulates your blood sugar and metabolic rate. Liver's nutritional value varies according to the type of animal and its diet, but as a general rule, a 100g serving of chicken, cow or lamb's liver contains well over 100 per cent of the recommended daily intake of vitamin A, which supports the immune system and is necessary for good skin, bones and eyesight (it helps you to see in the dark). In addition, liver and kidney meat from all sources, contain over 100 per cent of the recommended daily intake of vitamin B12, with calf's liver containing the highest concentration.

Liver also delivers significant doses of other B vitamins, including folic acid, riboflavin, B6, and niacin. Many of the nutrients found in liver are beneficial for cardiovascular health, but the downside is that it is high in cholesterol. A 100g serving of pan-fried calf's liver contains over 90 per cent of the safe daily limit. The level in chicken liver is higher, and in lamb's liver higher again. Since the liver is the organ that filters pollutants, I recommend eating livers from young, organic, grass-fed animals only, as they will have had less exposure to antibiotics, pesticides and hormones than those that have been intensively farmed. Organic liver also tastes better and is more tender in texture.

IMPORTANT NOTE: *In the UK, pregnant women are advised to avoid liver completely due to the high level of vitamin A, which can cause birth defects. If you have elevated cholesterol, seek your doctor's advice before including liver in your diet.*

Tips

- Liver is delicious fried with onions and herbs – fresh thyme is good – and a dash of balsamic vinegar.
- If the idea of eating a slice of liver does not appeal, chop it up and mix with minced beef to make a chilli con carne or bolognese sauce. This will add both richness and nutritional benefits to the sauce, while the herbs and spices will disguise the taste of the liver, if you do not like it.

10. Avoid commercially fried food

I didn't want to ban anything on my diet, apart from the additives detailed in previous sections – namely high-fructose corn syrup and trans and hydrogenated fats. This leads me to the subject of deep-fried food. I've always believed that 'a little of what you fancy does no harm', even if it means the occasional fast-food takeaway. But having read a great deal of the research into trans fats, I now avoid fried food in restaurants.

If you are in a country or one of the US cities or states where their usage is banned, then it is not so much of an issue. Otherwise, even in non fast-food restaurants, I avoid fries, as many French women do, most of the time. This is not just because they are fattening, but also because you cannot rule out the possibility that the restaurant has used cheap, partially hydrogenated oil for frying them. That such oils contain unsaturated fatty acids that become toxic when heated, is bad enough; but the fact that frying oil can be used and reused for several days – or in the worst cases, up to a week – means that the effect is magnified.

While chips and fried potatoes are the most common carriers of hidden trans fats, these artery-clogging fats can also be used to fry fish and meat. So unless a restaurant menu specifically states that a dish has been cooked in butter, or another fat that is stable and non-toxic when heated, I prefer to avoid fried food altogether, choosing grilled or braised meat wherever possible, when eating out.

Tips

- When ordering food in restaurants, always ask what kind of oil the food has been cooked in.
- Choose dishes where the meat or fish has been grilled or braised rather than fried.

PART FIVE

EXTRA STEPS TO IMPROVE YOUR DIET

The Marie Antoinette diet allows leeway for cake but central to this eating plan is the belief that taking small, positive steps to improve your overall diet, rather than focusing on negatives and things that you can't have, will also help with weight loss.

The more good stuff that you put into your body, the less you will crave the bad. So, in addition to the basic principles, I've added a few extra things you can do to boost your health and energy while following this diet.

1. Drink a glass of cucumber and celery juice daily

Although cucumbers were grown under glass in the kitchen garden at Versailles, Marie Antoinette did not, as far as we know, drink cucumber juice. But had she known about its benefits, she might have been persuaded. While fine-tuning my diet, I decided to include a daily glass of cucumber and celery juice for several reasons. Firstly, it's very hydrating – around 95 per cent water, in a form that is readily assimilated by the body – and it contains antioxidant polyphenols, along with reasonable amounts of vitamins K and C.

Cucumber juice also contains many alkaline minerals including calcium, phosphorus, potassium and magnesium, which help to counteract acidity in the body. What does this have to do with weight loss? Well, many practitioners of alternative medicine believe that an over-acidic system – caused by sugar, flour, vegetable oils, caffeine, alcohol, fizzy drinks, too much meat and processed food – is more prone to insulin resistance, and that it encourages the body to store the excess acid as fat in order to protect the major organs from the onslaught of toxins.

According to this theory,[50] it is important to make your body as alkaline as possible, not just for weight loss but for optimum health, since foods that are acid-forming when digested also leach important alkaline minerals such as magnesium, calcium and potassium in order to buffer or counteract the acid effect. Chronic over-acidity, it is said, corrodes body tissue and can increase the risk of auto-immune diseases such as osteoporosis and arthritis. I should point out that there is no supporting medical evidence[51] for the claims that an alkaline diet promotes good health, although the theory certainly sounds plausible. At the very least, strongly alkaline foods – avocados, leafy green vegetables, fresh figs, melons and green tea, for example – tend to be healthier choices than those that are very acid-forming such as sugar, flour, caffeine, vegetable oils and alcohol.

In traditional Chinese medicine, cucumber is also believed to have a detoxifying effect on the kidneys and liver. Given that certain organs such as the liver have to work harder to burn stored fat when you are on a diet, it seems to make sense to give your body a helping hand by feeding it 'clean' foods.

I first discovered the cleansing power of cucumber – juiced along with two sticks of celery, which is also very alkaline – at a detox retreat in Spain. We were given a large glass of cucumber and celery juice first thing, mid morning, after lunch and in the early evening, to cleanse, hydrate and alkalize the body. I hated the stuff but it's a habit that I've tried to continue at home, for as much as I dislike cucumbers, I find that this green juice helps to kill cravings for sugar and caffeine. It helps too, that you feel so virtuous after drinking it, that you think twice about chasing it down with toxins.

If you have a juicer, a glass first thing is a good way to start the day. No need to peel the cucumber, just wash it and shove it into the juicer with two sticks of celery.

Alternatively, drinking it in the evening will allow the juice to do its good work overnight. Either way, I find it helps to make it seem more glamorous if you think of actress Rene Russo drinking a glass of gloopy green juice to treat a hangover in *The Thomas Crown Affair*.

2. Chlorella

If you want to up the ante even more, you can add powdered chlorella to your green juice. Chlorella is an expensive and potent form of algae, which can make you feel nauseous if you are not used to it, so I recommend that you start with no more than half a teaspoon, if using the powdered form – the recommended intake for the pill form will be different – and increase your intake gradually. It is another of nature's secret 'superfoods', containing nine essential amino acids, as well as vitamins and minerals known to boost energy and help fight depression.

Chlorella is also rich in chlorophyll, which improves alkalinity and could potentially have an anti-inflammatory effect on the body. A 2013 study showed that chlorella can suppress histamine release, thereby reducing the body's inflammatory response,[52] although the study was carried out on rats and the benefits have yet to be proven in humans.

IMPORTANT NOTE: *Chlorella contains vitamin K1, which is a blood-clotting agent, so is not recommended for people taking warfarin.*

3. Add a spoonful of turmeric to soups and stews

Through the centuries this deep yellow spice has been used for many medicinal purposes, from the treatment of depression (in Chinese medicine) to afflictions of the skin, heart, liver and lungs (in Ayurvedic medicine). Preliminary research has started to back up some of these claims. Current studies suggest that it has anti-inflammatory properties and in high doses, may inhibit breast, colon and prostate cancers[53] as well as preventing the progression of Alzheimer's disease by removing amyloyd plaque build-up in the brain.[54]

For these reasons alone, it is worth finding ways to add the Indian spice to your diet. As far as weight loss is concerned, turmeric powder contains curcumin, which has been found to help increase the flow of bile, important for the breakdown of dietary fat. Wherever possible, I add a teaspoon of turmeric to any soups, stews, curries, and risottos that might benefit from its warm yellow colour.

IMPORTANT NOTE: *Pregnant women should consult their doctor before adding turmeric, as it can be a uterine stimulant.*

4. Stay happy by eating nuts and seeds

Adding nuts and seeds to your diet will help to provide the daily amount of magnesium that your body needs. Magnesium is the chill pill of the nutrient world since it calms the nerves and acts as an antidepressant, thereby contributing to the feel-good factor, which is an important aspect of this diet. It's also important for the metabolism of carbohydrate, as it influences the release of insulin, which means that it helps to control blood glucose levels and food cravings. In a 20-year study of nearly 5,000 people, those consuming the most magnesium in their diets were least likely to develop type 2 diabetes.[55]

Almonds, walnuts and Brazil nuts are all rich sources of magnesium, as are sunflower and pumpkin seeds. A daily helping of almonds – around 30g (1oz) – is one of the key recommendations of the Portfolio Diet. Created by Dr David Jenkins of the University of Toronto over a decade ago, this has been shown to lower levels of 'bad' cholesterol.[56]

I always keep a small stash of almonds with me – what the French call an *en-cas* – and find that a few teaspoons of nuts and seeds is a good mid-afternoon snack. Yes, I know what you're thinking: it sounds about as much fun as eating carrot batons. But nuts fill you up and they improve your mood. If really craving something sweet, you can add a few chocolate-coated Brazil nuts or raisins to the mix. It's better if you don't, but combined with the other nuts and seeds, this is still a better antidote to a sugar craving than a whole chocolate bar. Brazil nuts are also a good source of selenium, an antioxidant mineral.

5. Find a way to add linseed to your diet

Golden linseed, also known as flaxseed, is a nutritional powerhouse and a good source of essential fatty acids, which the body can convert into omega 3 fatty acids. Flaxseed is the dieter's friend because it is rich in both soluble and insoluble fibre, which helps to make you feel full. It doesn't taste too bad either: it has a nutty flavour and can easily be added to cereals or stews. I like to add a couple of teaspoons to a bowl of porridge, for a super-healthy snack.

You have to grind the seeds – easily done in a coffee grinder – as otherwise they will just pass straight through your body. Linseed also prevents constipation, which can be useful if you're on a diet.

IMPORTANT NOTE: *Linseed can aggravate some bowel and digestive tract disorders, so check with a doctor before adding it to your diet.*

PART SIX

LOSING ANOTHER FIVE
KILOS – MY STORY

Losing the first 5 kilos was fairly easy; the second 5 kilos, a little tougher but, following the steps that I've outlined in the previous section, it was still easier than I imagined. In the fifth week, as my diet evolved, I started to use bone broth as the base for all the soups that I made and noticed that, in addition to increased energy levels, my nails had never looked stronger. I also increased my repertoire of homemade cakes, so that when observing the evening fast, there was always something delicious to look forward to in the morning. This is very important, as boredom is the enemy of any diet. Eating cake early in the day, I noticed, also eliminated the desire for sweet stuff in the afternoon and evening.

The fact that there was no calorie counting at lunchtime also made it easier to stick to the regime, although I continued to keep a close eye on quantities, weighing out rice and pasta rigorously. I also acquired the habit of preceding lunch with a large salad, dressed with a teaspoon of melted coconut oil and balsamic vinegar, thus filling up with fresh vegetables and green leaves before the main course. The weight continued to fall off steadily, at between ½ to 1kg (1–2lb) a week – this despite the occasional dinner with friends, where I ate at least two courses, accompanied by wine.

I didn't feel guilty if broke the diet once or twice a week in this way. Instead, I reined it in the next day and chose one of the lowest calorie soups in my repertoire, such as the green broth (see recipe, p. 127) for dinner that evening. This degree of flexibility is important, as I'm convinced that rigid and prohibitive regimes are doomed to failure. Allowing yourself to take a couple of nights off in any given week, makes it easier, and less monotonous, to stick to the diet overall. In general, for the second five weeks of my diet, I ate soup and salad for dinner and observed an 8 pm food curfew for five nights out of seven. By the end of ten weeks, I'd reached my target weight.

Going forward

I'm by no means a 'skinny Minnie' but in ten weeks I lost enough weight – just under 10kg (1st 8lb) – to make a real difference. I now weigh 65kg (10st 3lb), which is not far off my former weight. My waist has also shrunk back to 81cm (32 inches) – safely below the diabetes danger zone of 89cm (35 inches).

Most importantly, I enjoyed the route that got me there. In creating this diet, I devised a way of eating that was tailor-made for me. This diet will work for others but each person needs to pick their pleasures wisely. Yours might be a glass of wine in the evening, in which case you need to make adjustments elsewhere – dropping the morning cake allowance, for example. It is about balancing the foods that give you the most pleasure with changes for the better, and slowly introducing new and healthier habits.

Losing weight the French way means realigning your attitude to food and accepting that every single thing that you eat affects your body in some way. When tempted to eat a chocolate bar after the 8.00 pm food watershed for example, I ask myself: 'What is this going to do for me?' and 'How is this going to make me feel?' Answer: in all likelihood, hungry for more. Conversely, when desperate for a mid-afternoon snack, don't look at a handful of almonds and think: 'How boring, I'd much rather eat a chocolate bar.' Instead, remind yourself: 'Almonds are rich in calcium and mood-boosting B vitamins and magnesium.

They are going to reduce my 'bad' cholesterol level, help lower my blood sugar and boost my brain function.'

I now try and apply the 'what will this do for me?' principle to almost everything I eat. That big plate of pasta? Most likely it will be followed by a huge energy slump and a second wave of hunger. This doesn't mean, 'don't eat pasta', but rather, 'moderate the quantity'. Remember that when you eat carbohydrates, like pasta, bread and cereals, the body metabolizes them as if they were sugar, although the rise in blood sugar varies according to the GI of the particular food.

Ultimately, you are the master or mistress of your calorific intake. One chocolate bar is not going to kill you; eating excessive amounts of sugar every day possibly will, in the long run. Once you've achieved your desired weight loss, the great thing about this diet is that if you feel the pounds creeping back on, you can redress the balance simply by replacing dinner or lunch with a bowl of soup and a salad. Do that just two or three times a week, and over a year that should add up to a lot of calories saved and kilos shed. As the French would say: *bon courage*.

The Marie Antoinette Diet summarized

1. You can eat cake but have it in the morning and no more than 75g (3oz).

2. If you are going to eat cake or baked foods, make them yourself – and reduce the recommended sugar content by at least 25 per cent.

3. Eat your main meal at lunch and make it as low GI as possible. If it's not practical to do this and dinner is your big meal, then eat soup or a salad for lunch instead.

4. Eat soup for dinner.

5. Try not to eat after 8.00 pm and observe a 12-hour fast from dinner to breakfast. (Do not do this if you suffer from diabetes or are hypoglycemic.)

6. Eat as little manufactured food as possible and always read labels. Avoid anything that contains hydrogenated fats, monoglycerides or diglycerides, monosodium glutamate or any kind of corn syrup.

7. Plan and shop ahead. Always make sure that there is something delicious waiting in the fridge when you get home in the evening.

8. Exercise portion control – of crucial importance for weight loss. If you are having pasta or rice for lunch, cut the serving back to 50–75g (2–3oz) dry weight, or 2 heaped tablespoons (100g or 4oz) cooked weight.

9. Rather than piling your plate high with carbohydrate, serve pasta, rice or other carb-based dishes in a small bowl and as the accompaniment to a large salad.

10. Eat liver once a week – 75–100g (3–4oz), raw weight, preferably organic.

11. Avoid bottled salad dressings, as they often contain sugar and undesirable additives. Instead make your own using melted coconut oil and balsamic vinegar. Alternatively, dress salads or vegetables with a teaspoon of olive oil and a little vinegar, or just a simple squeeze of fresh lemon or lime juice.

12. Keep a small bag or plastic tub (approximately 25g or 1oz) of nuts and seeds with you at all times for emergency food cravings and try and eat a couple of teaspoons of nuts and seeds a day.

13. Aim for variety. Dining Marie Antoinette-style or *à la française*, means eating a variety of small courses

at each meal, rather than a giant portion of one type of food. This makes meals more interesting and satisfying.

14. Boredom is the enemy of the dieter, so aim for variety in your overall diet by learning to cook at least one new dish every week.

15. Avoid cooking with vegetable oils. Instead, use coconut oil or butter wherever possible.

16. Avoid deep-fried or pan-fried food in restaurants, unless the dish has been cooked in butter. Especially avoid chips and French fries.

17. Only order dessert if it is amazing (and homemade).

18. Wherever possible, walk or do housework for 20 minutes after eating.

19. Keep up liquid intake – at least 1.5 litres of water every day.

20. Do not drink you sugar, be it in soft drinks, tea or coffee.

The 2-day Marie Antoinette Diet

The Marie Antoinette Diet was designed as a sensible and sustainable way of eating, resulting in longterm weight loss. Many of my French friends eat soup for dinner up to five nights a week, and for me the basic principle of this regime, of eating lightly in the evening, has now evolved into a long-term approach to food. However, for occasions when you do want a flatter stomach fast, the two-day plan below delivers results. It can also be used to kick-start a diet. Be sure to keep up fluid intake, by drinking at least 1.5 litres of water a day.

IMPORTANT NOTE: *The diet below should not be followed for more than two days. Do not do it if you are pregnant or are going to be very physically active.*

on rising (optional)

A glass of cucumber and celery juice – one whole, preferably organic, cucumber juiced with two stalks of celery.

breakfast

A small (80g or 3oz) portion of fruit with a plain, full-fat yoghurt and a teaspoon of chopped walnuts or other nuts sprinkled on top. Avoid high-sugar fruits such as banana and melon. Instead, any combination of blueberries, blackberries, strawberries or raspberries is ideal.

mid-morning snack

A small (75g or 3oz) piece of homemade cake or pastry – note the emphasis on small; this is meant to treat your taste buds, not sedate you – accompanied by a cup of green or herbal tea, or coffee.

lunch (your main meal)

STARTER: A bowl of soup (non-cream based).
MAIN COURSE: A small piece of protein such as chicken, salmon (tinned is fine), cottage cheese or a poached egg, accompanied by a large, colourful salad, dressed with either a teaspoon of melted coconut oil and a splash of balsamic vinegar, or a teaspoon of olive oil and a squeeze of fresh lemon or lime juice. The salad should contain at least five portions of raw vegetables and/or fresh salad ingredients.

afternoon snack

A handful (approx 25g or 1oz) of almonds mixed with pumpkin and sesame seeds. If craving something sweet, add half a dried fig or a couple of chocolate-coated Brazil nuts or raisins to the mix.

dinner

A bowl of bone or green broth (see recipe, p. 127) and a plate of vegetables (but not potatoes) dressed with lemon juice. Try not to eat later than 8.00 pm.

PART SEVEN

HEALING BROTHS

Bone broths are the ultimate in slow food. Traditionally, the way to make them is to stew bones for at least two hours, so that they soften and release their minerals into the stock. Some people add a tablespoon of vinegar or a splash of white wine to the cooking pot, as the acids are thought to help draw minerals from the bones.

A properly made bone broth has a gel-like consistency when it cools. This gel can be diluted with a little hot water to make a clear broth to drink straight up, or used as a base for other soups. It will keep for up to four days in the fridge and also freezes well. There are several variations of bone broth, including beef, lamb and chicken. I prefer to make the chicken version, and always use free-range, organic chicken in order to reduce exposure to pesticides and hormones. If you have a friendly butcher, you might be able to persuade him to give you bones for free.

CHICKEN BONE BROTH

Prep time: 30 mins + 2–4 hours cooking

Servings: 6–8 | Calories per serving: 108 kcal

*(based on 6 portions made with chicken pieces
with the meat still on the bones)*

It's ironic really, that something so delicious, and that many claim is so good for you, should be made from the bits of a chicken that would normally be thrown away. Traditional bone broth recipes feature chicken feet and necks, since the bonier parts of the bird are believed to make the most nourishing stock, with the tendons, bones and cartilage yielding glucosamine, chondroitin, collagen and trace minerals. Some believe that you should use as many tissue types as possible, including skin and fat, along with bone and ligaments. I couldn't quite handle the idea of chicken feet and other grisly bits, so I adapted the recipe to make it more user-friendly. The version that I make uses chicken legs, wings and thighs, with the meat still on them.

As for the meat that falls off the bones, you can either salvage it half way through the cooking process and use it for other dishes such as curries, stews or salads – it is very tender and a healthier option than fried meat – or add it back to the broth before serving in order to make a more substantial chicken soup.

In 18th-century Versailles, the cooks would have used the boiled meat from making bouillon, for delicious hors d'oeuvres or starters. Whatever you do with it, it is possible to generate several meals from this simple broth, if you make it from pieces of chicken with the meat still on the bone.

Alternatively, if you have cooked a roast chicken, you can use the leftover carcass to make bone broth. And after making the first batch, there is nothing to stop you from throwing the picked-clean bones back in the pot and starting all over again. In some cultures, it is quite normal to have a stockpot permanently simmering on the stove.

Many who swear by the broth drink a couple of bowls of it a day. Chicken bone broth makes an ideal base for other soups, stews and sauces, and can added by the spoonful to enrich other dishes. It can also be used instead of water when boiling rice, to add flavour.

Ingredients

1 whole carcass of a chicken *or*
2 free-range organic chicken
    thighs, 2 free-range organic
    chicken legs and/or breast
    bone and wings.
1 large onion
2 cloves of garlic
2 sticks of celery, chopped

2 large carrots
1 cup of kale or chard
1 organic stock cube or one
    teaspoon of Marigold
    bouillon powder
1 teaspoon of turmeric
herbs of your choice (I use
    thyme or fresh sage, which
    has detoxifying benefits)

Cover the chicken parts with at least 1 litre (1¾ pints) of water. Add the chopped onion, celery, garlic, turmeric and herbs, and simmer for at least 2 hours, topping up the water if necessary. When the meat is cooked and tender, normally after a couple of hours, remove it from the chicken bones and set aside. Strain the soup through a sieve to remove any bones or gristle and the stewed vegetables and then use a spoon to remove the fat that rises to the top of the bouillon. (Ideally, you should chill it in the fridge overnight, to allow the fat to solidify, as this will make its removal easier.)

The strained broth will cool to a jelly-like texture. I usually keep half of the cooled gel and freeze it to use in other soup recipes, and then return the other half to the pot to make chicken soup. To do this, dilute the gel with boiling water so that you have approximately 1 litre (1¾ pints) of liquid stock, then add the chopped carrot, along with the shredded chicken meat and the stewed vegetables set aside earlier. (Be sure that all bones and gristle have been removed.) At this point, if you feel that the soup needs more flavour, you can add the vegetable cube or powder. Simmer for a further 30 minutes and stir in the kale or chard in the last few minutes of cooking. (Instead of kale or chard, you could stir in Savoy cabbage or spinach just before serving, to further ramp up the nutrient value.)

BEEF BONE BROTH

Prep time: 10 mins + cooking time 6 hours
Servings: 6–8 | Calories per serving: 107 kcal
(based on 6 servings)

It can be difficult to source beef bones, even if you know a good butcher, as most meat is now cut into joints in processing plants. If you can find them, many people claim that beef bone broth is even more delicious, with more nutritional benefits, than the chicken version. The following recipe is reproduced with the kind permission of the Jade Institute, an oriental medicine school and wellness centre in Seattle, USA. There is more information, in addition to recipes for various bone broths at www.thejadeinstitute.com.

Ingredients

5–6 grass-fed beef bones, plus a large marrow bone (if available)

2 cups fresh kale, torn into bite sized pieces

3 carrots, sliced

½ cup green cabbage, sliced or chopped

1 cup chopped fresh parsley

2 shallot bulbs, chopped

5 cloves garlic, minced

½ –1 inch piece of ginger, minced

tablespoon of vinegar

herbs and seasonings as desired: choose from rosemary, fresh sage leaves

red pepper flakes, curry powder, Italian seasoning, tamari or soy sauce

Clean the bones and add to the pot with enough cold water to cover them. Bring slowly to the boil. Turn heat to low and add ginger, garlic, shallots, and vinegar. Cover and simmer for 6 hours. Allow to cool and place in refrigerator overnight for excess fat to congeal. On the day that you want to eat the soup, remove the pot from the refrigerator and use a large spoon to scrape off the top fat layer. Place the pot back on the stove and turn to medium-high heat. Add vegetables and spices. Cook at a simmer until ready to serve. Remove bones before serving.

GREEN (VEGETARIAN) BROTH

Prep time: 10 mins + cooking time

7 mins | Servings: 6

Calories per serving: 34 kcal

I cannot lie to you: this vibrant green vegetable broth is bland and frankly, rather a chore to eat. It tastes primarily of green beans. However, at 34 calories a serving, it is one of the best soups for weight loss. Its other big advantage is that, thanks to its high fibre content, it is very filling which means that you are less likely to resort to post-dinner snacks or give in to cravings.

It is based on a recipe by the late Dr Henry J Bieler, a prominent California-based physician who counted many 'motion picture stars' among his followers, including Greta Garbo, Lucille Ball and Gloria Swanson. One of the first doctors to pioneer a diet-based approach to health, Dr Bieler is best known for his book, *Food is Your Best Medicine*. This contains diet-based remedies for various diseases including diabetes, adrenal exhaustion and asthma, and although written in 1965, much of its advice is still relevant today.

The doctor was ahead of his time in many ways, recognizing the importance of diet for good health, and the negative effects of stimulants such as alcohol, sugar and caffeine on the adrenal glands. He was anti pharmaceuticals, believing that every drug, while remedying one problem, created a problem elsewhere in the body; and was convinced that better results could be achieved through 'the chemistry of food and the chemistry of the glands'.

In *Food is Your Best Medicine*, Dr Bieler lists the key ingredients for his healing vegetable broth – courgettes, runner beans, celery and parsley – but does not give precise quantities. There are many variations of 'Bieler broth' available on the Internet, but the recipe opposite remains faithful to the doctor's key ingredients and purist approach. Although you could liven up the broth by adding stock powder or seasoning, this would defeat Dr Bieler's original objective: he wanted to create a bland, restorative soup that would be as kind as possible to the kidneys and liver. (He believed that many illnesses, including arthritis, migraine, and cancer, were the result of 'acid intoxication' and the result of an overloaded liver.)

In addition to detox and weight loss, he recommended the broth for balancing the blood sugar and as an adrenal tonic for stress-induced conditions and fatigue. It contains minerals for restoring the acid-alkaline and sodium-potassium balance of the organs and for supporting the kidneys and liver.

Specifically, it contains vitamins C and K, folic acid, iron, fibre and calcium – nutrients that help to reduce the stress in your body and support adrenal health. Dr Bieler claimed that just one or two bowls of his broth would make a difference and deliver a significant health boost. All I can say is: try it for dinner one evening, and see how it makes you feel the next day.

Ingredients

4 cups (approx 600ml) of filtered water

3 stalks of celery, chopped

3 whole courgettes (zucchini)

2 cups of green string beans (frozen are fine if they are not in season)

1 small bunch of parsley, stems and leaves roughly chopped

2 cloves of garlic (optional)

pinch of dried oregano (not in Dr Bieler's original recipe but it makes the broth more palatable)

Pour 1 cup of water into a stockpot and steam the green beans above the boiling water for about 5 minutes. Then add the celery, courgettes and garlic and steam for 5 minutes or until tender, but still crisp. Do not overcook. Then put the steamed vegetables and the vegetable water, together with another 3 cups of water into the blender and liquidize. Add the parsley and a teaspoon of unsalted butter and blend again. The resulting broth can be quite thick, so you may need to dilute it with hot water (you can do this before each serving, if you prefer). The broth can be kept in the fridge for up to four days and also freezes well.

PART EIGHT

LET THEM EAT SOUP –
RECIPES FOR EACH SEASON

I tested many soup recipes while writing this book and found that certain soups suppress the appetite more than others; while some were just too much of a hassle to make. And so the criteria for inclusion were that the soup had to taste good, be easy to make, fill you up and provide nourishment – but not too many calories. Many of the recipes are based on so-called 'superfoods' – vegetables that have proven health benefits and are rich in antioxidants, thereby helping to protect against cancer and heart disease.

Although many of the recipes that follow suggest a tablespoon of olive oil for frying onions and other vegetables, I use virgin coconut oil wherever possible. Similarly, whenever stock is required I use bone broth instead of commercial stock cubes or powder, which boosts the health benefits of the soup. If you do use instant stock, I recommend Marigold Swiss Vegetable Bouillon powder in place of commercial stock cubes, as it is free from artificial flavourings and additives, and a low-salt version is also available.

AUTUMN

BROCCOLI SOUP

Prep time: 10 mins + 20 mins cooking
Servings: 6 | Calories per serving: 85 kcal

The beauty of this soup is that you use all parts of the broccoli, including the stalk, which is a good source of fibre. As green soups go, it is one of the most delicious, while broccoli needs no introduction as one of the world's healthiest foods. It is a good source of non-haem iron (that from a non-meat source) and antioxidants.

Ingredients

25g (1oz) butter for frying (less if you can get away with it)

1 medium onion, finely chopped

1 medium potato, chopped

350g (12oz) broccoli, including the stalk

900ml (1½ pints) vegetable or chicken stock

To serve (optional): a small cube of Gorgonzola, Roquefort or feta cheese crumbled into the soup before serving.

Melt the butter in a large saucepan and gently fry the onion and chopped potato for approximately 5 minutes. Add the stock and the chopped broccoli and simmer for a further 5–10 minutes until the potato is soft. Liquidize in a blender and then crumble in a small piece of cheese, if desired, before serving.

CARROT AND BUTTER BEAN SOUP

Prep time: 10 mins + 30 mins cooking
Servings: 6 | Calories per serving: 77 kcal

Carrot and coriander is the classic combination, but butter beans bring extra nutritional benefits to this soup – namely, potassium, magnesium, iron and protein – along with a rich creaminess and velvety texture. They're also a good source of soluble fibre, which is known to assist in lowering 'bad' LDL cholesterol.

Ingredients

15g (½oz) butter
150g (5½oz) onions, finely chopped
450g (1lb) carrots, grated
1 teaspoon ground coriander
225g (8oz) canned butter beans, rinsed and drained
1.2 litres (2 pints) vegetable or chicken stock
1 teaspoon of turmeric
2 tablespoons chopped fresh coriander
salt and black pepper
To serve: sprigs of fresh coriander

Melt the butter in a large saucepan, add the onions, and cook for approximately 5 minutes, until softened. Stir in the carrots and cook for a further 5 minutes. Add the butter beans and stock and bring to the boil. Then reduce the heat and simmer, covered, for 20 minutes or until the vegetables are tender. Remove the soup from the heat and liquidize. Stir in the chopped coriander and season to taste. Serve garnished with sprigs of coriander.

KALE AND CANNELLINI BEAN SOUP

Prep time: 5 mins + 10 mins cooking
Servings: 4 | Calories per serving: 144 kcal

If you think you are too busy to make your own soup, this one is for you. If you use pre-washed, bagged kale, it takes less than 5 minutes to prepare and 10 minutes to cook, and the ratio of nutritional value to effort is off the scale. Kale, which can be difficult to find in France and the UK, is one of the most powerful, but least recognized, greens. It contains a high concentration of beta-carotene, which the body converts to vitamin A, and is also a good source of vitamins C and K (important for bone health) and lutein, an antioxidant that promotes eye health.

When making this soup, add the kale at the last possible moment and 'flash' cook it for about a minute, until it is just past raw and turns a glossy shade of emerald. The shorter the cooking time, the more of the nutritional content you will conserve. I recommend organic kale if you can find it, while coconut rather than olive oil for the sautéing will enhance the flavour. Any leftover leaves can also be used to make salads, including a delicious modern twist on the Caesar salad, although it's a good idea to let the raw kale soften in the dressing for ten minutes or so before eating, as it can be quite tough.

IMPORTANT NOTE: *Anyone taking anticoagulants such as warfarin should consult their doctor before adding kale to their diet, because the vitamin K may interfere with the drugs.*

Ingredients

2 tablespoons non-virgin olive oil (or 2 teaspoons of coconut oil)

1 medium onion, chopped

100g (approx 4 cups of kale), chopped, washed and de-stalked

1 × 410g (14½ oz) can of cannellini beans, drained and rinsed

900ml (1½ pints) vegetable broth or stock

1 teaspoon turmeric

Heat the olive or coconut oil in a large saucepan. Add the onion and fry gently for 3 minutes. Pour in the stock, add the beans and the turmeric and let the mixture simmer for 5 minutes. Then stir in the kale, allowing it to cook for a couple of minutes until tender. Avoid letting it boil. Serve immediately.

SPLIT PEA SOUP WITH MUSTARD

Prep time: 20 mins + 55 mins cooking
Servings: 6 | Calories per serving: 238 kcal

Pea soup is one of the most comforting and filling soups you can make. There are many variations. Some people like to add chopped bacon or a ham bone for extra flavour, others a chopped carrot. The recipe below uses a teaspoon of Dijon mustard to pep up the taste, and give a warm, rich flavour. Sometimes I make an alternative version using a teaspoon of chopped fresh sage (which is believed to have an anti-inflammatory and anti-microbial effect) in place of the mustard and marjoram. You will need to soak the peas beforehand, preferably overnight.

Ingredients

375g (12oz) dried green split peas

15g (½oz) butter

½ teaspoon dried marjoram

1 teaspoon Dijon mustard

1 onion, chopped

900ml (1½ pints) vegetable or chicken stock

salt and pepper to taste

To serve: a small swirl of Dijon.

Soak the peas in cold water, for at least 4 hours. Drain and rinse well. Heat the butter in a large saucepan and fry the onion gently for 2–3 minutes. Add the peas, stock, marjoram and mustard. Bring to the boil; reduce to simmer and then cook, covered, for around 50 minutes until the peas are soft. Process the soup in a blender and season to taste. The soup is quite thick, so you might want to return it to the pot and add more stock or hot water before serving.

WINTER

LAMB AND GREEN BEAN SOUP

Prep time: 10 mins + 30 mins cooking
Servings: 4 | Calories per serving: 189 kcal

This substantial and filling soup is ideal for a cold winter night. It's a good idea to keep a couple of portions in the freezer for evenings when you return from work feeling ravenous. Although the recipe below suggests lamb neck fillet, I prefer to use lamb on the bone and cook it slowly (a minimum of 60 minutes) for maximum flavour and nutritional benefit. However, you must be careful to remove all fragments of bone before serving it.

Ingredients

1 teaspoon light olive oil
200g (7oz) lamb neck meat trimmed of fat and cut into cubes
½ large onion, finely chopped
50g (2oz) pearl barley
2 medium carrots, chopped
1 medium parsnip, chopped
3 teaspoons Worcestershire sauce
1 litre (1¾ pints) lamb or beef stock
2 thyme sprigs
110g (4oz) green beans (fresh or frozen), chopped

Heat the oil in a large saucepan and fry the lamb for a few minutes until brown. Add the onion and barley, and cook for a couple of minutes. Then add the carrots and parsnip and fry for 2 more minutes. Add the Worcestershire sauce, stock and thyme before covering and leaving to simmer for 30 minutes. When everything is cooked, and the lamb is tender, allow to cool slightly and remove any bone. Return the meat to the soup, then spoon about a quarter of it into a blender and process. Transfer from the blender back to the soup, add the green beans and simmer for a few more minutes until the beans are cooked but firm.

LENTIL SOUP

Prep time: 15 mins + 35 mins cooking
Servings: 8 | Calories per serving: 64 kcal

I played around with many lentil soup recipes before coming up with what I think is the winning formula. I use orange lentils as they not only bulk out the soup but give it a lovely golden colour, although you will need to soak them for 4–5 hours beforehand. Lentils are a good source of fibre, both the soluble kind, that helps to sweep up cholesterol in your blood, and insoluble. This little legume is also a good source of protein, magnesium and tryptophan, the precursor of the feel-good hormone serotonin, and it helps to stabilize blood sugar levels. So there you have it: a soup that is good for your heart and makes you happy.

Ingredients

1 teaspoon coconut oil (or olive oil) 1 medium onion, chopped

2 sticks of celery, chopped

1 medium carrot, chopped

100g (4oz) orange lentils (pre-soaked)

2 medium tomatoes, chopped

a few leaves of Savoy cabbage, chopped (optional)

1 litre (1¾ pints) chicken bone broth or vegetable stock

1 teaspoon turmeric

½ teaspoon ground cumin

Heat the oil in a large saucepan and add the onion, celery and carrot and fry for approximately 5 minutes until the onions are soft. Add the tomatoes, lentils and stock, along with the cumin and turmeric. Stir well. Cover and simmer until the lentils are cooked (approximately 30 minutes). Allow to cool slightly and then process in a blender. If the soup is too thick, you can add a little water before reheating. If you have made the soup with chicken bone broth rather than commercial stock, you might at this stage want to sprinkle in a little vegetable stock powder, depending on the taste.

SAVOY CABBAGE AND
CANNELLINI BEAN SOUP

Prep time: 5 mins + 20 mins cooking

Servings: 4 | Calories per serving: 114 kcal

A nourishing and filling meal in itself, this soup provides iron, fibre (especially the soluble form) and feel-good nutrients. Cannellini beans are low fat and a source of fibre. They also contain magnesium, some folate and the trace mineral molybdenum, which helps the body produce detoxifying enzymes.

Savoy cabbage meanwhile, contains phytochemicals, which act as antioxidants, boosting the immune system and helping to protect against breast, colon, and prostate cancers, as well as reducing 'bad' cholesterol in the blood. In short, it's hard to think of a more nutritious soup. The protein and fibre content will also keep you feeling fuller for longer, so that you are less likely to resort to snacks.

Ingredients

½ tablespoon light olive oil
3 garlic cloves, crushed
1 red onion, finely chopped
4 small carrots, finely sliced
2 courgettes, finely chopped
3 sticks of celery, finely chopped
1 × 410g (14½ oz) can of
   cannellini beans, rinsed and
   drained

600ml (1 pint) vegetable or
   chicken stock
1 teaspoon turmeric
200g (7oz) Savoy cabbage,
   shredded
25g (1oz) torn fresh basil leaves

Heat the olive oil in a large saucepan and then add the garlic, onion, celery, courgettes and carrots. Cook for 5 minutes, until the vegetables start to soften. Add the cannellini beans, stock and 100ml of boiling water. Bring to a simmer, stirring occasionally. Add the Savoy cabbage and cook for a further 5 minutes, until tender. Add a dash of freshly ground black pepper and stir in the freshly torn basil leaves before serving.

SPICY PARSNIP SOUP

Prep time: 10 mins + 35 mins cooking
Servings: 6 | Calories per serving: 121 kcal

Parsnips are a good source of potassium, folic acid and dietary fibre. This soup has anti-inflammatory properties thanks to compounds in the parsnips as well as the turmeric, onion and garlic. Coconut oil, if you have it, really enhances the spicy flavour. If you don't, you can use a light olive oil to roast the vegetables, instead.

Ingredients

4 teaspoons coconut oil
1 teaspoon coriander seeds
1 teaspoon cumin seeds
½ teaspoon ground turmeric
½ teaspoon mustard seeds
1 large onion, cut into 8 chunks

2 garlic cloves, peeled
675g (1lb 8oz) parsnips diced
1.2 litres (2 pints) vegetable stock
1 tablespoon lemon juice

Heat the oven to 200C/180C fan/400F/Gas 6. Melt the coconut oil in a metal roasting tin, on a low heat, on top of the oven. Then carefully mix in the spices, taking care to avoid spitting fat. Add the vegetables and mix well using a wooden spoon, so that the vegetables are coated in the oil and spread evenly over the tray, before putting it into the oven (use oven gloves as the tin will be hot). Roast for 30 minutes until the vegetables are tender; then transfer to a blender with half the stock and process until smooth. Pour into a pan with the remaining stock, season, and heat until barely simmering. Remove from the heat and stir in the lemon juice.

SPRING

SPRING VEGETABLE SOUP

Prep time: 15 mins + 25 mins cooking
Servings: 6 | Calories per serving: 68 kcal

This delicious multicoloured soup is full of fresh spring and early summer flavours and very nutritious. The leeks and courgettes make it a not insignificant source of iron, vitamin C, potassium, magnesium, folic acid and other B vitamins. It's worth using fresh mint and basil leaves if you can find them, as they really enhance the taste.

Ingredients

1 tablespoon olive oil
2 cloves garlic, minced
1 small onion, diced
1 leek, washed and thinly sliced
2 stalks celery, thinly sliced
1 courgette (zucchini) quartered
    lengthways, thinly sliced
2 medium carrots, halved
    lengthwise, then sliced

900ml (1½ pints) chicken or
    vegetable stock
1 teaspoon of turmeric
150g (6oz) frozen peas
1 teaspoon oregano
1 teaspoon dried basil
1 teaspoon dried thyme
shredded fresh mint leaves
torn fresh basil leaves

Heat the oil in a large saucepan over medium-low heat. Sauté the garlic, onions, celery, leeks and carrots for about 6–7 minutes, until softened. Add the courgette and sauté for another 2–3 minutes. Add the stock to the pan. Cover and bring to the boil. Reduce and simmer for 15 minutes. Add the peas and the dried herbs and stir for 1–2 minutes or until the peas are heated through. Season to taste and stir in the fresh herbs shortly before serving.

WATERCRESS SOUP

This wonderful, vitamin-packed soup is ideal for weight loss. It has even spawned its own slimming regime, the Watercress Soup Diet, which allows you to eat as much of it as you want. The soup, which is extremely low fat, became popular after actress Liz Hurley revealed that it was her fast-track route to a bikini body.

And where to begin with the wonders of watercress? Providing vitamins A (from beta carotene), B2, B6, C and E, this leafy green is nature's multivitamin. It also contains iron, potassium and iodine (needed for thyroid function), and a phytochemical that has been shown to inhibit breast, colon and prostate cancers. Prescribed by Greek physicians for numerous ailments as early as the 5th-century BC, watercress is also said to help redress viral infections, indigestion and high blood sugar.

I'm lucky to have a secret watercress source near my house in France, where in April and May, I can pick the lush green leaves from crystal clear water. During the watercress season, I make enough of this magical soup to last through the summer months and beyond, usually cooking and freezing it on the day that I pick the leaves, in order to preserve as much of the nutritional bounty as possible.

If you pick watercress in the wild, it's important to do so close to the source and ensure that it is from clean water, uncontaminated by animal droppings or other pollutants. You also need to know what you are looking for, as it is easy to confuse watercress leaves with poisonous water hemlock, which often grows nearby.

In the UK, one of the best suppliers of watercress is John Hurd, a Hampshire-based organic grower. The deep green leaves are in a different class to most supermarket watercress, and the peppery taste so potent that it feels almost medicinal. The raw leaf incidentally, is excellent for sore or tickly throats, and naturopaths recommend it as an expectorant if you have a cough or a cold.

I've included two different recipes for watercress soup below – the first is the slimming version with minimum fat, favoured by Liz Hurley; the second is slightly richer and more calorific. Whichever you choose, I recommend adding the leaves at the very final moment, cooking for no more than two minutes, and taking care not to boil them, in order to preserve as much of the vitamin C content as possible.

IMPORTANT NOTE: *Because of the high iodine content, this soup may not be suitable for people with hyperthyroidism (an overactive thyroid). Check with your doctor first.*

WATERCRESS SOUP I
THE SUPER SLIMMING VERSION

Prep time: 15 mins + 30 mins cooking

Servings: 6 | Calories per serving: 49 kcal

Ingredients

1 onion, finely chopped

1.2 litres (2 pints) of water or
  vegetable stock

2 small potatoes, peeled &
  chopped

3 large bunches of watercress,
  washed & de-stalked

To serve: a few watercress leaves
  and a swirl of plain yoghurt

Simmer the onion and potato in the stock until both are soft. Add the watercress and stir for 2–3 minutes. Remove from the heat and allow to cool slightly before processing in a blender. This version can be served hot or cold. To serve, swirl in a teaspoon of yoghurt and garnish with a few watercress leaves.

WATERCRESS SOUP II
THE LUXE VERSION

Prep time: 15 mins + 30 mins cooking
Servings: 4 | Calories per serving: 131 kcal

Ingredients

1 onion, finely chopped

25g (1oz) butter

250g (9oz) potatoes, peeled and
chopped

600ml (1 pint) chicken or
vegetable stock

2 large bunches (or 2 × 85g
bags) watercress, washed &
de-stalked

2 tablespoons natural yoghurt

a little milk if needed

salt and freshly milled black
pepper

To serve: a few watercress leaves
and a swirl of plain yoghurt

Melt the butter in a large pan and fry the onion until soft.
Add the potatoes and stock, and cook until the potatoes are
soft (approx 15–20 minutes). Then stir in the watercress,
'flash' cooking it for a couple of minutes. Remove from heat
and process in a blender until smooth. Then return to the
saucepan, adding a little milk or water if the soup seems too
thick. Add the yoghurt and seasoning. Serve hot, garnishing
each serving with a little extra yoghurt and some watercress leaves.

SUMMER

LETTUCE AND PEA SOUP

Prep time: 20 mins + 25 mins cooking

Servings: 4 | Calories per serving: 124 kcal

This is a lovely green summer soup and an ideal way to use up wilting lettuce leaves. Lettuce is particularly susceptible to pesticide residue, so wherever possible, this is one ingredient that you should buy organic.

Ingredients

25g (1oz) butter or coconut oil

1 large leek, trimmed and sliced

6 spring onions or one small onion, finely chopped

375g (13oz) Romaine lettuce, washed and leaves torn into pieces

900ml (1½ pints) vegetable or chicken stock

200g (8oz) peas (ideally fresh but frozen petits pois will do)

To serve: freshly chopped mint leaves or parsley

Heat the butter in a large pan and cook the leek and onions gently for 5 minutes. Add the stock and bring to the boil. Stir in the lettuce and peas and simmer gently for another 5 minutes. Remove from the heat and process in a blender until smooth. Serve with a sprinkling of chopped mint leaves or, if you prefer, parsley.

RED PEPPER AND PEAR SOUP

Prep time: 20 mins + 25 mins cooking
Servings: 4 | Calories per serving: 130 kcal

This is one of my favourite soups. It is bursting with anti-oxidants thanks to the carrot and peppers, which also give the soup its beautiful, deep red-orange colour. The peppers boost immune function and help to reduce inflammation in the body, as well as providing a good amount of lycopene, a vital antioxidant that is believed to help prevent cancers of the pancreas and prostate.

The pear adds sweetness and takes the sharp edge off the peppers; but in my opinion, it is the dollop of yoghurt and dash of hot Tabasco before serving that transforms this soup into something really special.

Ingredients

1 tablespoon olive oil
1 onion, chopped
1 large carrot, chopped
500g/ 3 large red peppers, de-seeded and chopped
750ml (1¼ pints) vegetable or chicken stock

1 large pear (approx weight 250g or 9oz) peeled and chopped
2 sprigs fresh thyme
salt and pepper
To serve: natural yoghurt and Tabasco sauce

Heat the oil in a large pan and gently fry the onion, peppers and carrot until soft (for about 10 minutes). Add the stock and bring to the boil. Add the pear and thyme; cover and simmer for about 25 minutes. Remove the sprigs of thyme and process the soup in a blender until smooth. At this stage you can pass the soup through a sieve to remove any pieces of pepper but it's not necessary. Season and serve with a swirl of natural yoghurt and a couple of dashes of Tabasco sauce.

VICHYSSOISE SOUP

Prep time: 15 mins + 15–30 mins cooking
Servings: 6 | Calories per serving: 55 kcal

French women regard vichyssoise as a five-star soup for weight loss and will eat nothing but leek soup for an entire weekend if they need to lose a few pounds. There are many variations of this classic French soup. Some people like to blend in fresh cream, British chef Jamie Oliver adds carrots to his, while in Provence they serve vichyssoise with chopped, hard-boiled egg on top. I'm a little more purist in my approach, but the version that I make can be served hot or cold. In France, this is *the* soup of summer.

Ingredients

1 knob of butter
2 medium leeks, finely sliced
225g (8oz) potatoes, peeled and cubed

1.2 litres (2 pints) chicken or vegetable stock
To serve: a swirl of plain yoghurt and chives

Melt the butter in a pan, add the leek and potatoes and cook until they start to soften. Add the stock, bring to the boil and simmer until the vegetables are soft. You can either serve it chunky or process in a blender for a smooth finish.

PART NINE

LET THEM EAT CAKE –
NUTRITIOUS AND DELICIOUS
DESSERT RECIPES

It might seem strange to include recipes for cake and cookies in a diet book, but my view is that if you are going to eat them, it is better to eat the homemade kind rather than the factory-produced. Also, sweet things can have nutritional value, especially if they contain nuts or fruit. I'm a big fan of ground almonds, which are not only very filling, so you eat less, but also rich in vitamin E, magnesium and mood-boosting B-complex vitamins.

The recipes below use less butter and sugar than comparable recipes but are delicious nonetheless. You can also play around with the ingredients, substituting coconut oil for a proportion (up to 50 per cent) of the butter, for example, to take advantage of the health benefits claimed for it. And remember: most desserts can be divided into portions and frozen, so that you are not tempted to scarf the lot at once.

CAKES

CHERRY ALMOND CAKE

Prep time: 20 mins + 30–35 mins cooking
Servings: 12 | Calories per serving: 215 kcal

Although I can't claim that this cake originates from Marie Antoinette's era – almonds did, however, feature strongly in 18th-century desserts – it is wonderful with coffee and takes less than twenty minutes to prepare. I use bottled black cherries from Lidl but you can also use glacé cherries or best of all, fresh black cherries, although halving and stoning them can double the preparation time.

Ingredients

100g (4oz) unsalted butter, melted
465g (1lb) cherries, fresh or canned, with the stones removed and cut in half
100g (4oz) plain flour
75g (3oz) ground almonds

1½ teaspoons baking powder
¼ teaspoon salt
2 large eggs
100g (4oz) caster sugar
1 teaspoon pure vanilla extract
80ml (3floz) whole milk
icing sugar for dusting

Preheat oven to 200C/180C fan/400F/Gas 6, and grease the bottom and sides of a 23cm/9″ springform tin. Melt butter and set aside to cool. In a bowl, mix together the flour, ground almonds, salt, and baking powder. Drain the canned or bottled cherries; or if using fresh cherries, remove the stones and halve the cherries before setting them aside. Using a hand blender, beat the eggs and sugar for about 5 minutes at high speed until thick and pale yellow; then stir in the vanilla extract.

Pour the butter and milk into the bowl, and then fold in the flour in three steps. Then add the cherries to the mix, gently folding them in. Pour the cake mix into the tin and even it out using a spatula. Place in the centre of the oven and bake for 30–35 minutes until golden brown. Leave on cooling rack for 15 minutes, and then remove the sides of the springform tin. Let it cool completely before removing the base.

CHOCOLATE AND COCONUT
SPELT CAKE

Prep time: 15 mins + 30–40 mins cooking
Servings: 12 | Calories per serving: 214 kcal

It's almost worth baking this cake just to fill your kitchen with the fabulous aroma of warm chocolate and coconut as it cooks. It's a cinch to make but quite rich to eat, so you only need a small slice. I use Green & Black's cocoa powder, which has a robust chocolaty taste. It has also been alkalized so that it has a neutral pH – natural cocoa powder is acidic – which makes it ideal for baking, as it does not alter the action of baking powder. Spelt is an expensive ingredient and can be difficult to find, but you can also make this cake with normal wheat flour (plain or self-raising, but if the latter, you won't need the baking powder) and still have a delicious homemade cake that is far healthier than supermarket offerings. You might find however, that you need to adjust the quantity. Using wheat flour, I find that the required amount is 4oz (100g).

Ingredients

150g (6oz) coconut oil

150g (6oz) caster sugar

2 eggs

4 tablespoons milk

75g (3oz) spelt flour

1 teaspoon baking powder

50g (2oz) unsweetened cocoa powder

To serve: dust with icing sugar (optional)

Preheat the oven to 180C/160C fan/350F/Gas 4 and grease and line a 20cm/8in sandwich tin. Place the coconut oil in a small dish and stand in a bowl of hot water until melted. Tip into a large bowl, add the sugar and beat together until combined. Then beat in the eggs, one at a time, before folding in the cocoa powder. Fold in the spelt flour and baking powder, alternating with the tablespoons of milk and making sure it is well combined. You should end up with quite a thick paste. Spread this mixture evenly in the cake tin and bake for 30–40 minutes, until it is shrinking away from the sides of the tin, or a knife inserted in the middle comes out clean. Leave to cool completely before removing from the tin.

LEMON YOGHURT CAKE

Prep time: 25 mins + 25 mins cooking
Servings: 8 | Calories per serving: 260 kcal

This is another great morning cake with a light, fluffy texture thanks to the yoghurt. I normally use spelt flour and add a teaspoon of baking powder to make it rise. (If you use spelt flour, you might find that you need slightly less – 150g rather than the 175g of self-raising flour cited below.) If you don't have coconut oil, you can replace it with butter but the combination of coconut oil and lemon is a match made in heaven. This cake also makes a good base for trifles.

Ingredients

1 lemon
50g (2oz) butter
50g (2oz) coconut oil
100g (4oz) caster sugar
2 eggs

160g (approx 2 small pots), plain yoghurt
175g (7oz) self-raising flour
½ teaspoon baking powder

Preheat oven to 180C/160C fan/350F/Gas 4. Grease a loaf tin and line with baking paper. Zest and juice the lemon, until you have approximately a tablespoon of each. Melt the butter and coconut oil in a saucepan or by standing in a small dish in a basin of hot water. Then using an electric whisk, beat the butter, coconut oil and sugar together in a bowl until pale and creamy. Add the eggs one at a time, followed by the yoghurt, lemon zest and lemon juice, beating until well mixed. Fold in the sifted flour and combine well. Then spoon the mixture into the prepared cake tin and smooth over the surface with a spatula. Bake for 20–25 minutes or until a skewer inserted in the centre comes out clean. Place on a wire rack to cool.

COOKIES

CHOCOLATE CHIP AND HAZELNUT
OAT COOKIES

Prep time: 15 mins + 15–20 mins cooking
Servings: makes 18 large cookies
Calories per serving/cookie: 189 kcal

These cookies are in a different league to the manufactured kind and thanks to the inclusion of porridge oats and nuts, bring many nutrients to the table, including B vitamins. The first time I made them I had to scrape them from the tin, as I had deliberately not greased it well enough. So, my advice is: do grease the cooking tray generously, and once they are out of the oven, gently work around the edges of each cookie with a palette knife to make it easier to remove them when they've cooled. You can, if you want to, substitute coconut oil for some of the butter – I use half and half – and if you prefer, use chopped walnuts or pecans instead of hazelnuts. These biscuits also freeze well.

Ingredients

125g (4½oz) butter, softened
200g (7oz) light brown, soft
   sugar
1 egg
1 teaspoon vanilla extract

75g (3oz) flour
¼ teaspoon bicarbonate of soda
125g (4½oz) porridge oats
65g (2½oz) chopped hazelnuts
90g (3½oz) chocolate chips

Preheat the oven to 170C/150C fan/325F/Gas 3. In a large bowl, beat together the butter and brown sugar until smooth. Beat in the egg and stir in the vanilla. Combine the flour and bicarbonate of soda, and stir into the creamed mixture. Then mix in the oats, hazelnuts and chocolate chips. Drop teaspoonfuls of the mix onto greased baking trays. Bake for 15–20 minutes and allow the cookies to cool for 5 minutes before transferring to a wire rack to cool completely.

FRUIT AND NUT COOKIES

Prep time: 15 mins + 10–15 mins cooking
Servings: 15 | Calories per serving: 176 kcal

Cookies containing oats and nuts have fibre and other nutritional benefits, so you don't have to feel quite so guilty about eating them. You can also tweak the recipe below, according to your favourite nuts and fruits.

Ingredients

50g (2oz) butter (melted)

50g (2oz) coconut oil (melted)

100g (4oz) soft brown sugar

1 egg

1 tsp vanilla extract

100g (4oz) self-raising flour

65g (2½oz) oats

50g (2oz) chopped hazelnuts

50g (2oz) desiccated coconut

50g (2oz) sultanas

Preheat the oven to 180C/160C fan/350F/Gas 4. Beat the sugar, coconut oil and butter together using a hand whisk. Add the eggs, one at a time, followed by the vanilla extract and a pinch of salt (optional). Stir in the flour, the oats, the coconut and sultanas, combining well. The mixture should form quite a stiff paste. Using a teaspoon drop the mixture onto a greased baking sheet (about two teaspoons for each cookie) patting down each one with the back of the spoon and leaving space for them to spread while cooking. Cook for 10–15 minutes or until golden brown.

GINGER NUTS

Prep time: 10 mins + 15–20 mins cooking
Servings: makes 15 biscuits | Calories per serving: 84 kcal

This is another quick and easy cookie recipe. Homemade ginger biscuits are far superior to the supermarket kind, and there are many health benefits associated with this lovely, warming spice. Numerous studies have shown that fresh ginger contains anti-inflammatory compounds, and can help with arthritis-related problems.[57]

Ingredients

50g (2oz) butter

50g (2oz) golden syrup (about 2 tablespoons)

40g (1½oz) soft brown sugar

175g (6oz) self-raising flour

2 teaspoons ground ginger

Preheat oven to 190C/170C fan/375F/Gas 5. Melt the butter, sugar and golden syrup in a pan until the sugar has dissolved. Blend with a balloon whisk until smooth. Leave to cool slightly, then sift flour and ground ginger into the sugar mixture and combine well. Form teaspoon sized amounts into small balls and arrange on greased baking sheets with plenty of space between them, as the mixture will spread. Flatten slightly using the back of a spoon, then bake in the centre of the oven for 15–20 minutes, until nicely browned. Transfer to a wire rack to cool completely.

WELSH CAKES

Prep time: 10 mins + 20 mins chilling + 6 mins cooking
Servings: makes 14 cakes | Calories per cake: 149 kcal

Less stodgy than a scone but more substantial than a cookie, Welsh cakes travel well and are a great snack to take to work. I make them with half butter and half virgin coconut oil, which also improves the texture. If you don't have coconut oil you can just double the amount of butter. The cakes keep well for up to a week in an airtight tin and also freeze well.

Ingredients

200g (7oz) plain flour

60g (2½oz) caster sugar

½ teaspoon mixed spice

½ teaspoon baking powder

50g (2oz) cold butter, cut into small pieces

50g (2oz) virgin coconut oil plus extra for frying

50g (2oz) sultanas

1 egg, beaten

splash of milk

Pour the flour, sugar, mixed spice and baking powder into a bowl. Using your fingers rub in the coconut oil and butter as if making pastry, until the mixture is crumbly. Then mix in the currants and work in the egg until you have a soft but not sticky dough. If the mixture seems too dry, add a little milk. Flatten the dough into a thick disc using your hands – you might find it easier to divide the mixture into two discs

– and leave in the fridge in a bowl covered with cling-film for 20 minutes. Roll out the dough on a lightly floured work surface, to a thickness of about ¾ of a centimetre and then cut out rounds using a 7cm (2.75″) crinkled, round cutter. Grease a flat griddle pan or heavy frying pan with coconut oil or butter and cook the cakes in batches on a medium heat, for about 3 minutes each side, until golden brown and cooked throughout.

DESSERTS

APPLE AND BLACKBERRY CRUMBLE

Prep time: 15 mins + 30–40 mins cooking
Servings: 8 | Calories per serving: 141 kcal

The great thing about fruit-based desserts is that they contribute to the all important five portions of fruit and vegetables per day (one serving of this pudding counts as half a portion of fruit). Blackberries are a valuable source of antioxidants. They're also economical to use as they can be picked from hedgerows and frozen, either whole or puréed. And if you have any leftover crumble mix, you can put it in a sealed plastic bag and freeze that for future use, too.

Ingredients

filling	topping
400g (14oz) apples	25g (1oz) unsalted butter, diced
1 teaspoon coconut oil	25g (1oz) coconut oil
2 teaspoons caster sugar	50g (2oz) caster sugar
100g (4oz) fresh blackberries	75g (3oz) plain flour
	25g (1oz) oats

Preheat the oven to 200C/180C fan/400F/Gas 6. Peel, core and chop the apples. Heat the coconut oil in a pan and sauté the apples gently, before adding the sugar. Stir until the apples are cooked, then add the blackberries and mix gently. For the topping, rub the butter and coconut oil into the flour and sugar until it resembles bread crumbs. Put the filling mixture into a shallow, 23cm/9in ovenproof dish and sprinkle the crumble mixture on top. Place in the oven for 15–30 minutes, until the topping is light golden brown and the blackberry juice is bubbling up at the sides.

PANCAKES

Prep time: 5 mins + 3 mins cooking
Servings: 4 | Calories per serving: 195 kcal

The beauty of pancakes is that they can be whipped up in minutes. With a history dating back to the 15th century, in France they are mostly eaten as a dessert, usually topped with a splash of Grand Marnier. You can increase the nutritional value by serving them with fruit, such as blueberries or bananas, and a little maple syrup, although I prefer them with a squeeze of lemon juice and a sprinkling of sugar.

Ingredients

100g (4oz) plain flour
1 large egg
275ml (½ pint) milk

20g (¾oz) coconut oil, melted, plus a little extra for frying
Lemon juice/sugar for sprinkling (optional)

Using a balloon whisk, blend the flour, egg, and milk together in a large bowl until you have a smooth mixture. Add the melted coconut oil and whisk again. Heat a little coconut oil in a small frying pan. When the pan is hot, pour in enough batter to make a thin pancake. Cook on one side until lightly browned then flip the pancake over and cook the other side. When cooked, add a liberal squeeze of lemon juice and sugar to taste, or serve with fruit.

ROSE-FLAVOURED RICE PUDDING

Prep time: 5 mins + approx 20 mins cooking
Servings: 6 | Calories per serving: 175 kcal

The 18th-century dessert menu relied heavily on milk-based puddings, such as blancmange, custard and cream-based ices. This Middle Eastern twist on a traditional rice pudding is a good dessert after highly spiced food. It's also super easy to make. Go lightly with the sugar – I suggest that you add a teaspoon at a time – as too much will ruin the delicate flavour. You can, if you wish, add a couple of drops of natural pink colouring.

Ingredients

500ml (18 fl oz) milk

25g/4–6 teaspoons of sugar (reduce to taste)

200g (7oz) white rice (basmati, risotto or any short grain rice) soaked for 20 mins

¼ teaspoon of cinnamon

a few drops of edible rose essence or up to 2 tablespoons of food grade rose water

To serve: chopped pistachios

Boil the rice in water until two-thirds cooked. Then drain the water and add the milk and cinnamon to the saucepan and bring to a boil over a gentle heat. Cook for 20 minutes or so, stirring occasionally, until the rice is soft and the milk is absorbed. (If the mixture becomes too sticky, add more milk.) Add the sugar in the last 5 minutes of cooking and finally, when the mixture is cooked, stir in the rose essence or rose water. (If you add it earlier, the heat tends to destroy the delicate flavour.) Then pour the pudding mixture into six ramekins and chill.

Below are some of the products and websites that I use and recommend, while doing this diet.

CHLORELLA

- Naturya Organic Chlorella Powder; www.naturya.com

CHOCOLATE/COCOA

- Green & Black's Organic Fairtrade Cocoa; www.greenandblacks.co.uk

COCONUT OIL

- Lucy Bee Fairtrade Organic Extra Virgin Coconut Oil; www.lucybee.co
  This is the oil that I use for cooking, baking and salad dressings. At the time of writing, the 300ml jar is available from Sainsbury's, £6.

SPELT

- Sharpham Park Organic Spelt Flour; www.sharphampark.com
  Also available from:
- www.planetorganic.co.uk
- Kilver Court Farm Shop, Kilver Street, Shepton Mallet, Somerset BA4 5NF; Tel 01749 340417; www.kilvercourt.com

ENDNOTES AND
RESEARCH PAPERS

1   Stéphanie Debette, Alexa Beiser, Udo Hoffmann, Charles DeCarli, Christopher J. O'Donnell, Joseph M. Massaro, Rhoda Au, Jayandra J. Himali, Philip A. Wolf, Caroline S. Fox and Sudha Seshadri. 'Visceral fat is associated with lower brain volume in healthy middle-aged adults'. *Annals of Neurology*, May 2010

2   The InterAct Consortium (2012). 'Long-term risk of incident type 2 diabetes and measures of overall and regional obesity': The EPIC-InterAct Case-Cohort Study. *PLoS Medicine*, 2012

    See also, Kathleen Doherty, www.diabetes.webmd.com, 'Waist size alone may predict diabetes risk', 5 June, 2012

3   James E. Brown, Michael Mosley and Sarah Aldred. 'Intermittent fasting: a dietary intervention for prevention of diabetes and cardio-vascular disease?'. *British Journal of Diabetes and Vascular Disease*, April 2013

4   Survey sponsored by dating website www.undercoverlovers.com.

    See also, Emily Payne, 'An affair "is better for weight loss than going on a diet"', *The Daily Mail*, 20 February 2013. http://www.dailymail.co.uk/health/article-2281600/Having-affair-good-waistline-libido.html#ixzz2Pm8TOoPD

5   *A Revolution in Taste: The Rise of French Cuisine, 1650–1800*, by Susan Pinkard (Cambridge University Press, 2010)

6   Campan, Jeanne-Louise-Henriette, *Mémoires de Madame Campan: Première Femme de Chambre de Marie Antoinette* (Mercure de France, 1999)

7   Shu-qun Shi, Tasneem S. Ansari, Owen P. McGuinness, David H. Wasserman and Carl Hirschie Johnson. 'Circadian disruption leads to insulin resistance and obesity', *Current Biology*, 21 February 2013. See also, news.vanderbilt.edu/2013/02/circadian-clock-obesity/

8   Jakubowicz D, Froy O, Wainstein J, Boaz M and E Wolfson. Med Center Tel Aviv University, Israel. 'Meal timing and composition influence ghrelin levels, appetite scores and weight loss maintenance in overweight and obese adults'. *Steroids*, March 2012

     See also: http://www.telegraph.co.uk/health/healthnews/9069276/Chocolate-cake-breakfast-could-help-you-lose-weight.html; 8th February 2012

9   Hatori M, Vollmers C, Zarrinpar A, DiTacchio L, Bushong E, Gill S, Leblanc M, Chaix A, Joens M, Fitzpatrick J, Ellisman M and Panda S. Salk Institute for Biological Studies, La Jolla, California, USA. 'Time-restricted feeding without reducing calorific intake prevents metabolic diseases in mice fed a high-fat diet'. *Cell Metabolism*, 2012

10   http://www.salk.edu/faculty/panda.html

11   Nils Halberg, Morten Henriksen, Nathalie Soderhamn, Bente Stallknecht et al. 'Effect of intermittent fasting and refeeding on insulin action in healthy men'. *Journal of Applied Physiology*, June 2005

12   http://www.northwestern.edu/newscenter/stories/2011/05/night-owls-weight-gain.html

13   Julie E. Flood and Barbara J. Rolls. Pennsylvania State University, USA. 'Eating soup preloads in a variety of forms reduce meal energy intake'. *Appetite*, 14 April, 2007

14   Rolls BJ, Bell EA, Thorwart ML. 'Water incorporated into a food but not served with a food decreases energy intake in lean women'. *American Journal of Clinical Nutrition*, 1999

15   'How Soup Can Help You Lose Weight,' by Jack Challoner. http://news.bbc.co.uk/2/hi/uk_news/magazine/8068733.stm

16   LeSauter et al. 'Stomach ghrelin-secreting cells as food-entrainable circadian clocks'. *Proceedings of the National Academy of Sciences*, 2009

17 George Cheyne, *An Essay of Health and Long Life*, 1745

18 Brownell K, Gold M. 'Food products. Addiction. Also in the mind'. *World Nutrition*, September 2012

19 Volkow N.D, Wang G.J, Tomasi D, and Baler R.D. 'Food and drug reward: overlapping circuits in human obesity and addiction'. *Behavioral Neuroscience*, 2012

   See also: http://www.bnl.gov/medical/RCIBI/Research/obesity.asp

20 *Salt, Sugar, Fat: How The Food Giants Hooked Us*, by Michael Moss. (WH Allen, 2013)

21 http://www.dailymail.co.uk/news/article-2066737/Only-ONE-meal-home-cooked---thats-30-cent-drop-eighties.html

22 Helen Lawson, 'Only one in six mothers cooks from scratch each day because they lack time and confidence in the kitchen', *The Daily Mail*, 8 March 2013

   http://www.dailymail.co.uk/news/article-2290106/Only-mothers-cooks-scratch-day-lack-time-confidence-kitchen.html#ixzz2Q9wfFb8X

23 Source: the Obesity charity MEND

24 Gayaneh Kyureghian, Rodolfo M. Nayga, Jr., George C. Davis, Biing-Hwan Lin. 'Obesity and food away from home consumption by restaurant type and meal occasion: can fast food and lunch away from home make you fatter?' *International Journal of Obesity*, December 2007

25 Almudena Sánchez-Villegas, Estefania Toledo, Jokin de Irala, Miguel Ruiz-Canela, Jorge Pla-Vidal, Miguel A Martínez-González. 'Fast-food and commercial baked goods consumption and the risk of depression.' *Public Health Nutrition*, 2011

26 Mozaffarian D, Pischon T, Hankinson SE, et al. 'Dietary intake of trans fatty acids and systemic inflammation in women.' *American Journal of Clinical Nutrition*, 2004

27 Mozaffarian D. 'Trans fatty acids – effects on systemic inflammation and endothelial function'. *Atherosclerosis Supplements*, May 2006

28. Kavanagh K, Jones, KL, Sawyer J, Kelley K, Carr JJ, Wagner, JD, Rudel LL. 'Trans fat diet induces abdominal obesity and changes in insulin sensitivity in monkeys'. *Obesity*, May 2007

See also: 'Six years of fast-food fats supersizes monkeys'. *New Scientist,* June 2006

29 Source (re countries that have banned trans fats): http:// en.wikipedia.org/wiki/Trans_fat

30 Enig, Dr Mary and Fallon, Sally, *Eat Fat, Lose Fat: The Healthy Alternative to Trans Fats* (Hudson Street Press, 2005)

31 Katz DL, Evans MA, Nawaz H, Nkike VY, Chan W, Comerford BP and Hoxley ML. Yale Prevention Research Centre, USA. 'Egg consumption and endothelial function: a randomized controlled crossover trial.' *International Journal of Cardiology*, 2005

32 Valentine Njike, Zubaida Faridi, Suparna Dutta, Angelica L Gonzalez-Simon and David L Katz. Yale Prevention Research Centre, USA. 'Daily egg consumption in hyperlipidemic adults – effects on endothelial function and cardiovascular risk'. *Nutrition Journal*, 2010

33 Michael A Roussell, Alison M Hill, Trent L Gaugler et al. Pennsylvania State University, USA. 'Beef in an Optimal Lean Diet study: effects on lipids, lipoproteins, and apolipoproteins'. *American Journal of Clinical Nutrition*, January 2012

34 Dr Roussell quoted in the *Daily Mail*, 5 March 2013. http://www. dailymail.co.uk/health/article-2288088/Steak-After-warnings-saturated-fat-unhealthy-hearts--Stop-feeling-guilty-that-juicy-steak-good-you.html

35 Forette B et al. 'Cholesterol as risk factor for mortality in elderly women'. *The Lancet*, 1989

36 M Garaulet, P Gómez-Abellán, J J Alburquerque-Béjar, Y-C Lee, J M Ordovás and F A J L Scheer. 'Timing of food intake predicts weight loss effectiveness'. *International Journal of Obesity*, 29 January 2013

37 University of Copenhagen Faculty of Life Sciences. 'The dark chocolate version of Father Christmas is most filling'. October 2008 http://www.life.ku.dk/English/Nyheder/2008/965_dark_ chocolate.aspx

38 Lesley L Moisey, Sita Kacker, Andrea C Bickerton, Lindsay E Robinson, and Terry E Graham. 'Caffeinated coffee consumption impairs blood glucose homeostasis in response to high and low glycemic index meals in healthy men'. *American Journal of Nutrition*, May 2008

See also: 'Coffee and croissant – the enemies of weight loss', by Patrick Holford, www.patrickholford.com, 9 March, 2009 http://www.patrickholford.com/index.php/blog/blogarticle/314/

39 Miriam E. Bocarsly, Elyse S. Powell, Nicole M. Avena, Bartley G. Hoebel. Princeton Department of Psychology and Princeton Neuroscience Institute, USA. 'High-fructose corn syrup causes characteristics of obesity in rats: increased body weight, body fat and triglyceride levels.' Published online by Pharmacology, *Biochemistry and Behaviour*, 26 February, 2010

40 Professor Hoebel quoted in www.princenton.edu online article, 'A sweet problem: Princeton researchers find that high-fructose corn syrup prompts considerably more weight gain,' by Hilary Parker, 22 March 2010 http://www.princeton.edu/main/news/archiveS26/91/22K07

41 M Garaulet, P Gómez-Abellán, J J Alburquerque-Béjar, Y-C Lee, J M Ordovás and F A J L Scheer. 'Timing of food intake predicts weight loss effectiveness'. *International Journal of Obesity*, 29 January 2013

42 *Napoleon and Josephine: An Improbable Marriage*, by Evangeline Bruce. (Weidenfeld & Nicolson, 1995)

43 'Bone and vegetable broth,' by RA McCance, W Sheldon and EM Widdowson. The Biochemical and Children's Departments, King's College Hospital, London, 1934. Available to read at www.adc. bmj.com

44 Mahmood A. Aljumaily. Department of Surgery, College of Medicine, University of Mosul, Iraq. 'The effect of concentrated bone broth as a dietary supplementation on bone healing in rabbits'. *Annals of the College of Medicine*, Mosul, volume 37 No. 1 & 2, 2011

45 Rennard BO, Ertl R, Gossman G, et al. Pulmonary and Critical Care Medicine Section, Nebraska Medical Center, Omaha, NE. 'Chicken soup inhibits neutrophil chemotaxis in vitro'. *Chest*, October 2000

46 Maria D. Guillén, Patricia S. Uriarte. Faculty of Pharmacy, University of the Basque Country, Spain. 'Aldehydes contained in edible oils of a very different nature after prolonged heating at frying temperature: presence of toxic oxygenated, unsaturated aldehydes'. *Food Chemistry*, April 2012

47 Assuncao ML, Ferreira HS, dos Santos AF, Cabral CR Jr, Florencio TM. Faculdade de Nutrição, Universidade Federal de Alagoas, Maceió, Brazil. 'Effects of dietary coconut oil on the biochemical and anthropometric profiles of women presenting abdominal obesity'. *Lipids*, July 2009

48 Chinmay Manohar, James A. Levine, Debashis K Nandy, Ahmed Saad et al. Mayo Clinic, Rochester, Minnesota. 'The effect of walking on postprandial glycemic excursion in patients with type 1 diabetes and healthy People'. *Diabetes Care*, 8 August 2012

49 This recipe was featured in *Le Cuisinier Gascon*, by Louise Auguste de Bourbon a cookery book written in 1740 and quoted in *Savoring the Past, The French Kitchen and Table from 1300 to 1789*, by Barbara Ketchum Wheaton, (Touchstone, 1996)

50 *The pH Miracle: Balance Your Diet, Reclaim Your Health*, by Dr Robert O Young and Shelley Redford Young (Piatkus, 2009)

51 Tanis R Fenton, Suzanne C Tough, Andrew W Lyon et al. 'Causal assessment of dietary acid load and bone disease: a systematic review & meta-analysis applying Hill's epidemiologic criteria for causality'. *Nutrition Journal*, April 2011

52 Min-Jung Bae, Hee Soon Shin, Ok Hee Chai, Jae-Gab Han, Dong-Hwa Shon. 'Inhibitory effect of unicellular green algae (Chlorella vulgaris) water extract on allergic immune response'. *Science of Food and Agriculture*, published on-line, 5 April 2013

53 'Fighting cancer at your local Indian restaurant by eating curry'. www.sciencedaily.com, 2 March 2011 http://www.sciencedaily.com/releases/2011/03/110302101744.htm

54 Shrikant Mishra and Kalpana Palanivelu. 'The effect of curcumin (turmeric) on Alzheimer's disease: an overview'. *Annals of Indian Academy of Neurology*, January–March, 2008

55 Jia-Yi Dong, Pengcheny Xun, Ka He and Li-Quiang Quin. 'Magnesium intake and risk of type 2 diabetes: meta-analysis of prospective cohort studies'. *Diabetes Care*, September 2011

56 'David J. A. Jenkins et al. 'Effect of a Dietary Portfolio of Cholesterol-Lowering Foods Given at 2 Levels of Intensity of Dietary Advice on Serum Lipids in Hyperlipidemia. A Randomized Controlled Trial'. *Journal of the American Medical Association*, August 2011

See also: 'Portfolio Diet: Recipe for Lower Cholesterol'. www.
webmd.comhttp://www.webmd.com/cholesterol-management/
features/portfolio-diet-lower-cholesterol

57 Wigler I, Grotto I, Caspi D, Yaron M. 'The effects of Zintona EC
(a ginger extract) on symptomatic gonarthritis'. *Osteoarthritis
Cartilage*, November 2003

FURTHER READING

DIET AND NUTRITION

Bieler, Henry J, *Food is Your Best Your Medicine* (Ballantine Books Inc; reissue edition, 1996)

Enig, Dr Mary and Fallon, Sally, *Eat Fat, Lose Fat: The Healthy Alternative to Trans Fats* (Hudson Street Press, 2005)

Moss, Michael, *Salt, Sugar, Fat: How The Food Giants Hooked Us* (WH Allen, 2013)

Shanahan, Catherine MD, *Deep Nutrition: Why Your Genes Need Traditional Food* (Big Box Books, 2008)

The Weston A Price Foundation; www.westonaprice.org
This US nonprofit organization aims to educate the public in the 'wise traditions' of food and farming. The website contains lots of inspiring nutrition advice.

MARIE ANTOINETTE AND THE HISTORY OF FRENCH CUISINE

Campan, Madame, *Mémoires de Madame Campan, Première Femme de Chambre de Marie Antoinette* (Mercure de France, 1999)

De la Varenne, Pierre Francois, *Le Cuisinier François: D'après l'édition de 1651* (Editions Manucius, 2003)

Feydeau, Elisabeth, *Jean-Louis Fargeon, Parfumeur de Marie Antoinette* (Perrin, 2004)

Pinkard, Susan: *A Revolution in Taste: The Rise of French Cuisine, 1650–1800* (Cambridge University Press, 2009)

Weber, Caroline: *Queen of Fashion: What Marie Antoinette Wore to the Revolution* (Aurum Press, 2007)

Wheaton, Barbara Ketchum, *Savoring the Past, The French Kitchen and Table from 1300 to 1789* (Touchstone, 1996)

ACKNOWLEDGMENTS

The quotations from *Eat Fat Lose Fat: The Healthy Alternative to Trans Fats*, in the section entitled 'Marie Antoinette did not eat trans fats, margarine or low-fat spreads,' are reproduced with the kind permission of the authors Dr Mary Enig and Sally Fallon. *Eat Fat Lose Fat* is an eye-opening and inspirational read, that I would recommend to anyone seeking to lose weight.

Thank you also to Dr Susan Pinkard, who not only gave me permission to quote from her book, *A Revolution in Taste: The Rise of French Cuisine, 1650–1800*, but generously corrected some of the assumptions that I had made about the 18th-century diet at Versailles.

The recipe for beef bone is reproduced with the kind permission of The Jade Institute, www.thejadeinstitute.com in Seattle, USA.

I'd like to thank the Facebook group LIFT (Ladies in France Together), and the French members especially, for sharing with me their weight loss tips.

Thank you to Lucy Bee Limited, for allowing me to reproduce the pancake recipe from www.lucybee.co, where you can find many other delicious recipes using the brand's Fairtrade, organic coconut oil.

Big thanks to my friends in the blogosphere for giving me and/or my books space on their blogs.

And an enormous, general merci to my two favourite *Françaises*, Martine Mousserion and Patti Huisse.

AUTHOR BIOG

Karen Wheeler lives in France and is a former fashion editor of the *Mail on Sunday* newspaper. As a freelance writer she wrote regularly for the *Financial Times How To Spend It* magazine for over a decade. Her work has also appeared in the *Daily Mail*, *The Times*, *Sunday Times Style*, *You* magazine and numerous international publications. She is also a three-time winner of the Jasmine literary award for writing about fragrance. Updates of her daily life in France can be found on her blog, www.toutsweet.net and on Twitter.com as @mimipompom1.

Other books by this author:

Tout Sweet: Hanging up My High Heels for a New Life in France

Toute Allure: Falling in Love in Rural France

Tout Soul: The Pursuit of Happiness in Rural France

INDEX

Note: Page references for recipes are in **bold**